Fortschritte der
Urologie und Nephrologie

Vem goer sa att stjaernorna lyser,
som jag i dina oegon ser?

(Wer bringt die Sterne zum Leuchten,
die ich in deinen Augen seh?)

Eva Dahlgren

Hans-Peter Schmid

The clinically organ-confined adenocarcinoma of the prostate

Natural history, selection criteria for radical prostatectomy and prognostic factors based on long-term follow-up

Steinkopff Darmstadt

Dr. Hans-Peter Schmid
Urologische Klinik
Universität Basel
Spitalstraße 21
CH-4031 Basel

Die Deutsche Bibliothek – CIP-Einheitsaufnahme

Schmid, Hans-Peter:
The clinically organ confined adenocarcinoma of the prostate : natural history, selection criteria for radical prostatectomy and prognostic factors based on long term follow-up / Hans Peter Schmid. – Darmstadt : Steinkopff, 1994
(Fortschritte der Urologie und Nephrologie ; 28)
ISBN-13: 978-3-7985-0998-6 **e-ISBN-13: 978-3-642-85430-9**
DOI: 10.1007/ 978-3-642-85430-9
NE: GT

ISSN 0071-7975

Medical Editorial: Sabine Ibkendanz – English Editor: James C. Willis – Production: Heinz J. Schäfer

Typesetting: Typoservice, Alsbach
Printed on acid-free paper

Preface

Dr. Hans-Peter Schmid has addressed in this monograph the basic dilemmas surrounding prostate cancer. These dilemmas include the 40 % histologic incidence of invasive cancer in men in comparison to a 3 % death rate, the extraordinary slow doubling time of four to five years for untreated early clinical stages (T1 and T2 cancers), the limited life span of even healthy men over 70 years of age, and the national and international debates of how to treat this cancer.

It is important, however, to recognize that despite these uncertainties, prostate cancer is probably the most predictive of all human solid tumors. Dr. Schmid has addressed the basis for much of this predictability in this monograph. The level of serum PSA and its rate of increase in the untreated patient with a prostate size of less than 50 grams is undoubtedly the most useful of all measurements in predicting volume and grade of the cancer, but it is closely followed by assessment of the extent and percent of grade 4 and 5 cancer in six systematic, spatially separated biopsies. Estimating the amount of suspected cancer on digital rectal examination by assigning a clinical stage is useful, but far less quantitative than PSA and systematic biopsies.

The Basel series in this monograph adds strong support to these basic concepts.

April 1994

Thomas A. Stamey, M.D.
Professor and Chairman
Department of Urology
Stanford University School of Medicine
Stanford, California, USA

Contents

I. Introduction and overview

1.1 Historical remarks

Prostatic diseases as a problem of the elderly man have already been mentioned in the Ebers-papyrus from 1500 B.C. In 1817 Langstaff for the first time differentiated between benign and cancerous tumors of the prostate (Herbst and Polkey, 1933).

Surgical treatment for prostate cancer started in 1866 and 1867, respectively when Kuechler and Billroth performed the first perineal prostatectomies (Kuechler, 1866; Murphy, 1972). At the beginning of this century it was Young (1905) at Johns Hopkins University who systematically developed the technique. However, high incontinence rates prevented the operation from becoming generally accepted.

Renewed interest in prostate surgery started in 1945 through the introduction of the retropubic approach (Millin, 1945). Finally, the nerve-sparing retropubic radical prostatectomy developed by Walsh and coworkers (Walsh and Donker, 1982; Walsh et al., 1983) has greatly increased the number of radical prostatectomies performed in the United States.

1.2 Epidemiology

Prostate cancer is now the most common of all male cancers (except for skin cancer) in Western countries and second only to lung cancer in mortality (Boring et al., 1993). In the United States, 165'000 newly diagnosed cases are estimated for 1993 and 35'000 men will eventually die from prostate cancer (Boring et al., 1993). Among all races in the United States, the age-adjusted mortality rate from prostatic adenocarcinoma established for 1983 to 1984 is 22.7 deaths per 100'000 men, and the incidence is 75.3 cases per 100'000 men (Devesa et al., 1987). Although it is mainly a disease of older men, it is estimated that a death from prostate cancer represents, on average, 9.0 years of life lost (Horm and Sondik, 1989).

1.3 Etiology

Environmental, familial and endogenous factors have been studied in order to identify etiologic or predisposing factors for prostate cancer (Carter et al., 1990; Scardino, 1989). There are only a few established risk factors for the development of clinically apparent prostate cancer, namely increasing age, race and a positive family history. Prostate cancer is very uncommon before the age of 50 years, but its frequency climbs steeply with age to peak or plateau in the 9th decade for both incidence and mortality rate (Lew and Garfinkel, 1990). Blacks in the United States have a mortality rate for prostate cancer that is two to three times the rate for whites in the same geographic area, even when it is corrected for socioeconomic status and age (Ernster et al., 1977). However, the frequency of incidentally found prostate cancer at autopsy was similar between the two races (Guileyardo et al., 1980). In this study and in another smaller series (McNeal et al., 1986), the proportion of incidental cancers that were large and poorly differentiated was considerably greater in blacks than in whites. Several sources have documented the familial aggregation of prostate cancer (Cannon et al., 1982; Spitz et al., 1991; Steinberg et al., 1990a; Woolf, 1960). A two to threefold increase in risk has been reported for men having a father or brother with clinical carcinoma of the prostate, and the relative risk may exceed five if two or more first-degree relatives have had clinical prostate cancer (Steinberg et al., 1990a). The same investigators provided evidence that prostate cancer is inherited in mendelian fashion, at least in a subset of families (Carter et al., 1992a).

Despite much research efforts in the field of molecular and cellular biology and early encouraging reports on the role of certain oncogenes in prostate cancer (Viola et al., 1986), currently no oncogenes (Peehl, 1993) or structural chromosome aberrations (Breitkreuz et al., 1993) have been correlated conclusively with the initiation or progression of this type of cancer. The situation seems to be similar for tumor-suppressor genes (Bookstein and Allred, 1993).

The hormonal hypothesis in the etiology of prostatic cancer is supported by the discovery of steroid hormone receptors in prostatic carcinoma and by the ability to manipulate prostate cancer growth rates through hormonal therapy. Furthermore, Noble (1977) was able to increase the incidence of prostate cancer in Nb rats through chronic administration of testosterone and estrogen. However, the results of several studies have been conflicting or negative, and it has been proposed that the role of androgenic hormones is only a permissive one (Carter et al., 1990).

Several other factors have been discussed in the carcinogenesis (cadmium, increased dietary fat intake, sexually transmitted infectious agents) or prevention (beta-carotene, retinoid, vitamin D) of prostate cancer (Skowronski et al., 1993; Zaridze and Boyle, 1987). Recently, the relationship between vasectomy and prostate cancer has been widely disputed but still remains unclear (Giovannucci et al., 1993a; Giovannucci et al., 1993b; Nienhuis et al., 1992).

1.4 Diagnosis

1.4.1 Primary diagnostic tests

The increased incidence of prostate cancer is the result of several factors including increased awareness among clinicians and the public of the significance of carcinoma of the prostate, the aging of the population, and improvements in diagnostic methods. For many decades, diagnosis of prostate cancer has relied on digital rectal examination (DRE) and digitally guided biopsies or fine needle aspiration (FNA). In population studies this combination had a detection rate of only 0.8 to 1.7 % (Chodak et al., 1989; Scardino, 1989).

Currently, three primary diagnostic tests to initiate histologic or cytologic tissue sampling are useful in making the prostatic cancer diagnosis: DRE, prostate-specific antigen (PSA) and transrectal ultrasonography (TRUS). The significance of prostatic induration or nodularity during DRE is well recognized. However, already in 1956 Jewett found that only approximately 50 % of lesions palpated by the clinical examination and considered suggestive of carcinoma actually were malignant on biopsy (Jewett, 1956). More recent analyses have further diminished the value of DRE. In a review of 15 series based on abnormal DRE findings, 795 of 2073 (38 %) perineal needle biopsy specimens detected carcinoma (Hodge et al., 1989b). The same authors noticed that in five series of transrectal biopsies done on 728 patients, 322 samples (44 %) contained carcinoma. In a morphometric study, McNeal and colleagues (1988) could demonstrate that only 44 % of prostate tumors were located on the rectal surface and accessible to DRE (Figure 1). Moreover, the same group found a broad range of tumor volumes within given clinical stages (Spigelman et al., 1986). Finally, in a case-control study, screening by routine DRE appeared to have little if any effect in preventing metastatic prostate cancer (Friedman et al., 1991).

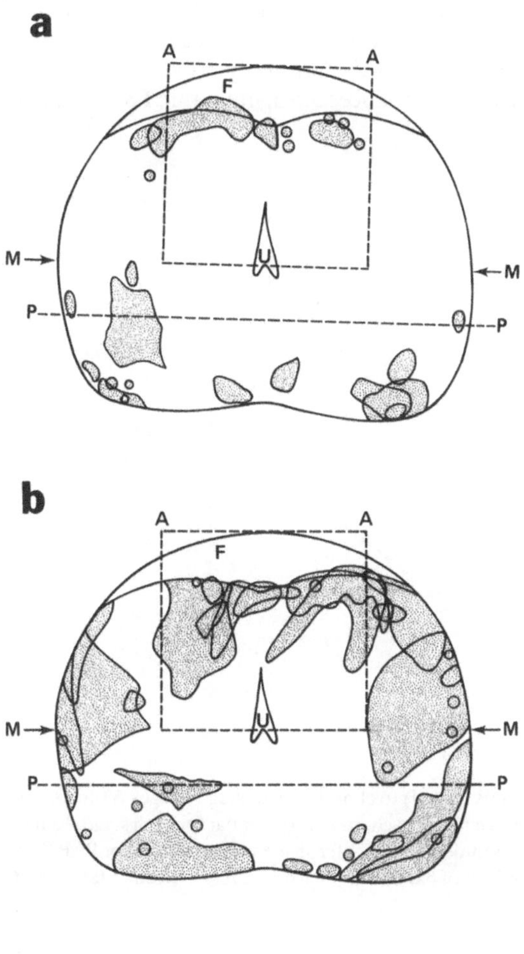

Fig. 1. a transverse plane through mid portion of prostate shows locations of 25 small incidental carcinomas from cystoprostatectomy for bladder cancer. **b** locations of 38 small carcinomas found unexpectedly as additional independent primary tumors in prostates removed for adenocarcinoma. U, urethra. M, midline of glandular prostate. F, fibromuscular stroma. Within box A-A, zone of stage A cancers. Posterior to line P-P, zone of stage B cancers (from: McNeal et al., 1988).

After several years of clinical experience, PSA appears to be the best overall serum marker for prostate cancer and may be the best tumor marker in all of cancer biology. PSA is a kallikrein-like serum protease with a molecular weight of 33'000 to 34'000 daltons that is produced exclusively by the epithelial cells of the prostate gland. Using immunoelectrophoretic analysis Sensabaugh first characterized this "semen-specific protein" and called it p30 (Sensabaugh, 1978). Later, at Roswell Park, Wang et al. (1979) isolated an antigen from prostatic tissue, purified it and demonstrated its specificity with prostatic tissue. In 1990 Graves and coworkers concluded that PSA and the semen protein p30 were identical and could be easily purified by a rapid continuous technique (Graves et al., 1990a). Different commercially available assays for the determination of PSA in serum make its comparison somewhat difficult and prompted the need for an international antigen standard (Graves et al., 1990b). For more detailed information on PSA see the excellent review article by Oesterling (1991).

For clinical purposes, PSA proved to be superior to prostatic acid phosphatase (PAP) in assessing clinical stages (Stamey and Kabalin, 1989). As depicted in Figure 2, serum PSA is proportional to increasing clinical stage, whereas serum PAP fails to distinguish the increasing cancer volume associated with clinical stages B1, B2 and B3. Moreover, serum PAP of patients with stages A1, A2 and B1 is within the normal range of PAP for patients without prostate cancer. Apart from clinical stages, the Stanford group was also able to demonstrate a proportional relationship between serum PSA and the volume of benign prostatic hyperplasia (BPH) and prostate cancer, respectively. On average, 1 gram or 1 cc of BPH produces 0.3 ng/ml serum PSA as measured by the Yang polyclonal assay (Stamey et al., 1987) and 1 gram or 1 cc of prostate cancer produces 3.5 ng/ml serum PSA (Stamey

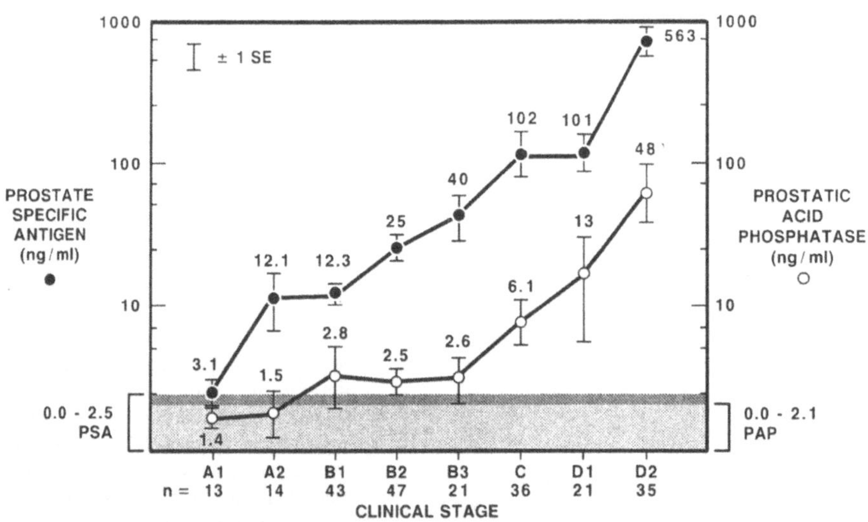

Fig. 2. Relationship of PSA and PAP concentrations (ng/ml) to clinical cancer stage (stages A1 to D2) in 209 patients. Mean values of PSA and PAP are shown above each standard error bar for each stage. Range of serum PSA for normal subjects (0 to 2.5 ng/ml) is indicated by lighter shaded area and that for PAP (0 to 2.1 ng/ml) is shown by darker shaded area. n, numbers of patients in each clinical stage (from: Stamey and Kabalin, 1989).

et al., 1989). These data have been confirmed by others (Partin et al., 1990; Perrin et al., 1991). Catalona and his group used PSA as the initial test in an early detection program. They concluded that the combination of serum PSA and DRE, with TRUS performed in patients with abnormal findings, provided a better method of detecting prostate cancer than DRE alone and that PSA is the most accurate of the three tests for this purpose (Catalona et al., 1991). The author's opinion on how to interpret PSA and DRE as the primary diagnostic tools for detection of early prostate cancer and when to initiate TRUS-guided biopsies is based on the natural history of prostate cancer and is delineated in chapter 2.5 of this thesis.

TRUS has emerged as the most common approach for imaging the prostate. In 1971, Watanabe et al. published the results of size and volume measurements of the prostate and, in 1975, suggested its utility in staging and monitoring prostate cancer (Watanabe et al., 1975). Today the state-of-the-art TRUS machine uses real-time imaging with a 7-MHz transducer and has the capability for both transverse and sagittal imaging of the prostate. Early enthusiasm for TRUS as a staging tool for prostate cancer has diminished, since it is not capable to identify microscopic disease (Rifkin et al., 1990). Furthermore, due to its relatively low sensitivity and specificity and its cost TRUS does not seem indicated for early detection of prostate cancer if both PSA and DRE are normal. Probably TRUS is best used to guide the needle biopsy (Brawer, 1993).

In 1989 Hodge and coworkers introduced the technique of random systematic ultrasound guided transrectal core biopsies of the prostate (Hodge et al., 1989b). This method has substantial advantages over the conventional directed hypoechoic biopsies. Apart from a considerable nonspecificity of hypoechoic lesions for cancer (Lee et al., 1989) the six systematic biopsies can yield information on the spatial distribution of cancer in relation to potentially positive surgical margins and can better estimate the overall histological grade of the whole tumor. Furthermore, TRUS guided biopsies performed by the random-systematic technique potentially provide the most information about tumor volume (Hammerer et al., 1992; Hodge et al., 1989b).

Finally, there is a subset of 10 – 20 % of patients whose cancer is detected incidentally at transurethral resection or open prostatectomy for presumably benign prostatic hyperplasia (Brawer, 1993).

1.4.2 Additional examinations

The measurement of serum acid phosphatase and the increased serum levels associated with advanced prostatic carcinoma were first described by Gutman and Gutman (1938). For decades serum enzymatic acid phosphatase was the standard marker for prostate cancer until Foti and colleagues (1975) introduced an immunologically specific radioimmunoassay (RIA) for prostatic acid phosphatase. RIA-PAP proved to be much more sensitive and reproducible than enzymatic assays (Heller, 1987; Huber et al., 1982). However, with knowledge of serum PSA neither enzymatic nor RIA-PAP can yield additional information for the detection (Brawer, 1990; Huber et al., 1987) or staging (Burnett et al., 1992; Stamey and Kabalin, 1989) of localized prostate cancer and, thus, should be abandoned.

The results of computerized tomography (CT) and magnetic resonance imaging (MRI) for preoperative staging have been disappointing (Mukamel et al., 1986). Both modalities fail to appreciate microscopic extraprostatic disease, which is far from the resolving power

(Rifkin et al., 1990). CT as well as MRI have a low sensitivity of identifying small lymph node metastases (Hammerer et al., 1992). The development of endorectal probes for MRI has increased the sensitivity in detecting extraprostatic disease, but the high costs and expense make its routine clinical use doubtful (Hering and Mueller, 1991; Schnall et al., 1989).

In clinical use for 30 years now, radionuclide bone scan (BS) is the most sensitive method to detect skeletal metastases (Schaffer and Pendergrass, 1976). The role of BS in newly diagnosed, untreated prostate cancer patients with low serum PSA levels has been evaluated by Chybowski et al. (1991). They found that in 306 men with a serum PSA of 20 ng/ml or less (Hybritech assay) only 1 had a positive BS (negative predictive value 99.7 %) and concluded that a staging radionuclide BS in a previously untreated patient with a serum PSA in that range may not be necessary. However, one has to bear in mind that those patients were referred to the Mayo Clinic for radical prostatectomy and therefore were a highly selected group.

Cystoscopy and intravenous urograms are not necessary in the evaluation of clinically localized prostate cancer unless the patient has microscopic hematuria. Lymphangiography and vesiculography are completely obsolete nowadays. In summary, none of the above mentioned additional examinations – with the possible exception of BS – is mandatory for staging prostate cancer prior to radical prostatectomy.

1.5 Staging and grading

As outlined in the preceeding chapter 1.4. staging of prostate cancer prior to radical prostatectomy is based on PSA, DRE, random systematic TRUS guided biopsies and – perhaps still – BS. The present thesis deals with clinically organ-confined tumors; two different staging systems were used. The patients in the Basel series were clinically and pathologically staged according to the TNM-system from 1987 (Hermanek and Sobin, 1987) (Table 1). We were well aware of the potential disadvantages of this system. For example, invasion of the apex of the prostate is categorized together with extracapsular disease as T3 rather than T2 (organ-confined). The patients in the Stanford series were staged according to the modified Whitmore-Jewett classification (Jewett, 1975; Whitmore, 1956) (Table 2). Stage B cancers were further substaged into B1, B2 and B3 (Stamey and Kabalin, 1989) (Figure 3).

The distribution of clinical stages at time of diagnosis of prostate cancer has been documented best by a population-based study from Sweden (Johansson et al., 1989). In a restricted geographic area, all men (n = 654) with newly diagnosed prostate cancer underwent radionuclide BS, chest radiography, and intravenous urography. The clinical stages of prostate cancer on initial presentation are shown in Table 3. Overall, only 47 % of all tumors were clinically organ-confined at time of diagnosis. However, Donohue et al. (1982), Gervasi et al. (1989) and Smith et al. (1983) could demonstrate that in this group of clinical T1-2 NX M0 (A-B) tumors 30 % had already positive pelvic lymph nodes, thus reducing the number of pathologically confined cancers to at most one third in the general population. Of the patients with clinical stage T3 NX M0 (C), 50 % are known to have lymph node metastases (Donohue et al., 1982; Zincke et al., 1986).

The grading system most generally used in the United States is the Gleason system (Gleason, 1977; Gleason et al., 1974). This grading system was defined and validated by

Table 1. TNM staging system 1987 (Hermanek and Sobin, 1987)

Primary tumor			
TX	Primary tumor cannot be assessed		
T0	No evidence of primary tumor		
T1	Incidental carcinoma	T1a	3 foci or less
		T1b	more than 3 foci
T2	Palpable tumor, confined to the gland	T2a	1.5 cm or less in diameter
		T2b	more than 1.5 cm or involving more than one lobe
T3	Palpable tumor, invasion of prostatic apex or beyond the prostatic capsule or bladder neck or seminal vesicle; not fixed		
T4	Tumor is fixed or invades adjacent structures other than those listed in T3		
Regional lymph nodes			
NX	LN cannot be assessed		
N0	No LN metastasis		
N1	Metastasis in a single LN, 2 cm or less in diameter		
N2	Metastasis in a single LN, more than 2 cm but not more than 5 cm diameter; or multiple LN, none more than 5 cm in diameter		
N3	Metastasis in a LN more than 5 cm in diameter		
Distant metastases			
MX	Presence of distant metastasis cannot be assessed		
M0	No distant metastasis		
M1	Distant metastasis		

the follow-up data on 2911 patients. It was standardized with a simple line drawing (Figure 4) and is based solely on architectural criteria. Cytologic abnormalities are not considered in this system because they tend to parallel the architectural changes quite closely. There are five histologic grades in the Gleason system (Figure 4). A "primary" grade is assigned to the pattern occupying the greatest area of the specimen and a "secondary" grade to the pattern occupying the second largest area. Primary and secondary grades are added to

Table 2. Modified Whitmore-Jewett Staging System (Jewett, 1975; Whitmore, 1956)

A		Incidental carcinoma
	A1	focal
	A2	diffuse or poorly differentiated
B		Palpable tumor, confined to the gland
	B1	focal
	B2	diffuse
C		Palpable tumor, beyond the prostatic capsule
	C1	minimal extracapsular extension
	C2	extensive extracapsular extension
D		Distant metastases
	D1	Pelvic lymph node metastasis
	D2	Bony or other distant metastasis
	D3	Hormone resistant stage D2 (relapse after endocrine therapy)

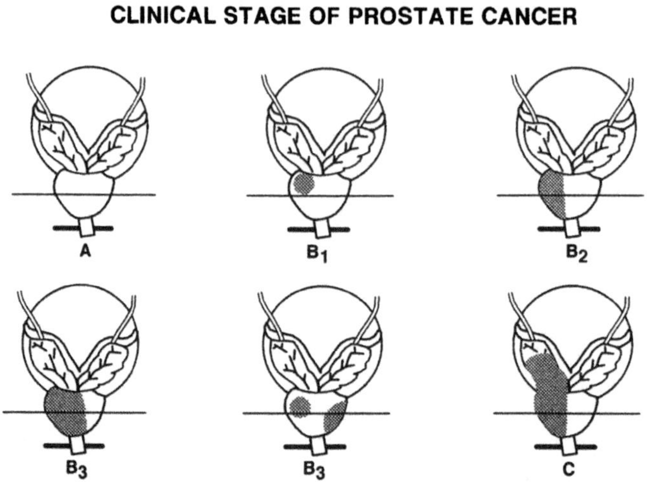

Fig. 3. Clinical staging criteria for prostate cancer based on digital rectal examination for clinical stages A, B and C disease: stage A – incidental or unsuspected cancer; stages B1 and B2 – unilobar palpable nodules but stage B1 must not extend for greater than length of half of 1 lobe; stage B3 – bilaterally palpable disease; stage C – extension into 1 or both seminal vesicles, or extension outside posterolateral capsule (from: Stamey and Kablin, 1989).

give a "score" (range 2-10). From the original data of Gleason (1977) it can be concluded that the distribution between grade 3 or better (score 6 or better) versus grade 4 or worse (score 7 or worse) makes the greatest prognostic impact on the greatest number of patients. This distinction is superficially a distinction between well differentiated carcinoma and poorly differentiated carcinoma.

The grading system mostly used in Switzerland and Germany is the Dhom system (Dhom, 1977; Mueller et al., 1980). It assignes only three different histological grades: grade 1 (well differentiated), grade 2 (moderately differentiated) and grade 3 (poorly differentiated). In comparison to the Gleason system, grade 1 corresponds roughly to Gleason score 2-4, grade 2 to Gleason score 5-7 and grade 3 to Gleason score 8-10.

Table 3. Clinical stages of prostate cancer at time of diagnosis (n = 654)

T1 NX M0	A	17 %
T2 NX M0	B	30 %
T3 NX M0	C	28 %
T1–4 NX M1	D2	24 %
		99 %

(adapted from Johansson et al., 1989)

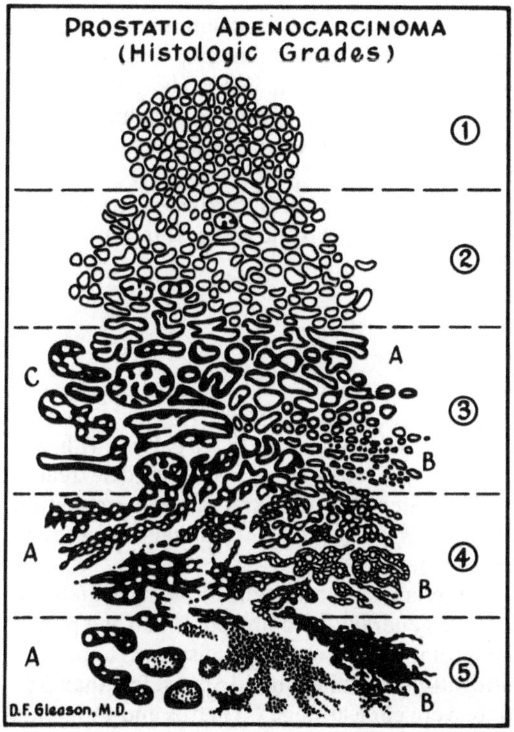

Fig. 4. Diagram illustrating the histologic pattern of each Gleason grade and also the sub-classification within grades (from: Gleason, 1977).

1.6 Treatment options

1.6.1 Deferred treatment (wait and watch)

In Great Britain and Scandinavia especially, the general policy toward newly diagnosed prostate cancer is to defer treatment until symptoms occur. Favorable outcome has been reported for clinically localized cancer by Adolfsson and Carstensen (1991), George (1988) and Johansson and colleagues (1989). In a smaller, retrospective analysis, Stenzl and Studer (1993) came to similar conclusions. However, these series were highly selected since the majority of histological grades were well differentiated (G1), the age of the patients was fairly advanced and a considerable number of patients received some sort of therapy.

Whitmore and associates (1991) retrospectively reviewed 75 patients with clinical stage B prostate cancer who received no therapy for at least one year after diagnosis. For stage B1, B2 and B3 lesions, median follow-up was 124, 120, and 96 months, respectively and actuarial survival at 15 years was 67 %, 39 %, and 63 %, respectively. They observed that the first evidence of tumor progression was usually local and that all cancers were apparently growing, albeit at potentially slow rates.

The Veterans Administration Cooperative Urological Research Group (VACURG) has conducted the only prospective randomized trial comparing radical prostatectomy versus placebo (Madsen et al., 1988). After 15 years there was no significant difference in cumulative survival between the surgically treated and the non-treated patients. For some good reason this study has been critisized (Voges and Hohenfellner, 1990). There was only a small number of patients randomized and the drop out rate was 22 %. Staging at study entry was crude and follow-up was not well defined. Finally, the exact cause of death was unknown.

Clearly, assessing the life expectancy of patients with prostatic carcinoma prior to the decision of who should be treated, how should they be treated and when is far more important than for any other genitourinary malignancy.

1.6.2 Radical prostatectomy and radiotherapy

In the United States, Switzerland and Germany there is consensus that a patient with clinically localized prostate cancer and a life expectancy of ten or more years should be treated with curative intent. For many years, radical prostatectomy and external beam irradiation have been considered equally effective (Bagshaw et al., 1988; National Institutes of Health consensus development conference, 1987).

Although the indications for radical prostatectomy for carcinoma of the prostate have changed significantly over the past decade, one generally-held precept is that the preferred patient for this procedure is one in whom total extirpation of the disease is to be anticipated (clinical stages A and B). At major institutions in the United States, less than 1 % of patients undergoing radical prostatectomy were clinical stage C (Petros and Catalona, 1992; Quinlan et al., 1991; Stamey et al., 1989). However, there are some advocates of radical prostatectomy for limited clinical stage C disease when supplemented with immediate adjuvant bilateral orchiectomy or radiation (Zincke et al., 1986). The clinical dilemma is even worse for patients, in whom frozen sections of pelvic lymph nodes reveal cancer or in whom permanent histologic sections were positive (stage D1). The question is whether to proceed with radical prostatectomy to achieve local control (Steinberg et al., 1990b), to combine radical prostatectomy with immediate hormonal therapy (Zincke, 1989), to combine radical prostatectomy with delayed hormonal therapy (deKernion et al., 1990), or to leave the prostate in situ and treat with radiation or hormonal therapy. Currently, palliative radical prostatectomy to achieve local control in clinical stages C and D1 seems not to be justified (Schroeder, 1991).

In prostate cancer found incidentally at transurethral resection or simple prostatectomy for presumable BPH, many suggestions have been made to separate those patients who need further treatment from those who can be followed (Kastendieck, 1984). Most subclassifications into stage A1 and A2 are based on the percentage of tumor in the resected chips. For prediction of prognosis in the individual patient these subclassifications remain insufficient. Lowe and Listrom (1988) could demonstrate that in clinical stage A prostate cancer tumor volume and Gleason grade of the resected tumor were consistently related to progression. The linear relationship of tumor volume and serum PSA (Stamey et al., 1989) prompted Voges and associates (1992b) to evaluate the predictive value of serum PSA levels at least four weeks after TURP for substantial residual cancer volume. They found that 19 of 20 patients with a PSA level of more than 2.5 ng/ml (Yang assay) had more than 0.9 cc of cancer, whereas seven of eight patients with less than 1.0 ng/ml PSA had a residual volume of less than 0.4 cc. They concluded that only patients with PSA levels below 2.5 ng/ml and negative TRUS-guided modified systematic biopsies (Terris et al., 1992) need no definite treatment.

In their large series of more than 900 patients Bagshaw et al. (1988) reported excellent results of external beam irradiation for clinically localized prostate cancer. However, of great concern is the high positive biopsy rate after radiation therapy. After 18 months or more 61 % of patients undergoing finger-guided, perineal biopsies had cancer in the sample (Freiha and Bagshaw, 1984). At a mean of 5.2 years after radiation therapy 93 % of patients were positive for cancer when systematic TRUS-guided needle biopsies were performed (Kabalin et al., 1989). The majority of these biopsy-positive patients harbor biologically active disease and will subsequently develop metastases (Freiha and Bagshaw, 1984; Schellhammer et al., 1987).

Recently we have presented the longest follow-up to date on serial PSA levels after irradiation (Stamey et al., 1993b). Eighty-eight of 113 patients (78 %) had a precipitously rising PSA at a mean follow-up of five years after radiotherapy. Twenty-three patients (20 %) appear cured with a stable serum PSA below 1.7 ng/ml (Yang assay) at a mean follow-up of nine years. Two of the 113 patients (2 %) continue to have a falling PSA three years after therapy. Clinicopathologic documentations of failure are generally preceeded by an increase in PSA levels during follow-up (Ritter et al., 1992). From these data we conclude that only about 20 % of patients with clinical stages A-D1 prostate cancer can be cured by irradiation therapy.

In a prospective randomized study Paulson and associates (1984) found no difference in the time to first evidence of distant metastases in patients randomly assigned to external beam irradiation and those expectantly treated with delayed androgen deprivation at time of metastases.

There are a few reports comparing radical prostatectomy to radiation therapy. In a retrospective analysis, Ziegler et al. (1990) found that surgery was superior to radiation with regard to tumor progression and tumor-related survival. The only prospective randomized trial comparing the two treatment modalities was conducted by Paulson et al. (1982). Eighty months after therapy 75 % of radical prostatectomy treated patients and 48 % of radiation treated patients were free of disease. With regard to long-term follow-up, survival after 10 years was better in radical prostatectomy series when compared to radiation series (Frohmueller et al., 1991).

1.6.3 Hormonal therapy and chemotherapy

Although advanced prostate cancer is not the topic of this thesis, I shall briefly discuss the main issues of palliative treatment to complete the overview. At least two thirds of all patients have nonorgan-confined disease at time of diagnosis (chapter 1.5.) and, thus, are not amenable to curative treatment. They will eventually be faced with local problems (Schmid, 1991) and/or distant metastases.

Since the Nobel prize-winning demonstration of hormone dependency of prostatic cancer by Huggins and Hodges (1941), suppression of testicular androgens has remained the most effective palliation for patients with advanced disease with rates of retarding tumor growth in 70 to 80 % of the cases (Altwein, 1982; Ruebben and Altwein, 1987). In the field of hormonal therapy, two significant clinical issues must be addressed. First, should therapy be started immediately upon recognition of an incurable stage of prostate cancer or can it be delayed as long as the patient remains asymptomatic? Second, should only testicular androgens be withdrawn or should androgens produced by the adrenal glands also be suppressed?

For more than 20 years, most clinicians have followed the recommendations of the Veterans Administration Cooperative Urological Research Group that therapy "... be withheld until the patient's symptoms were so severe as to require relief" (VACURG, 1967a; VACURG, 1967b). However, Sarosdy (1990) has reanalyzed the data of these studies and came to the conclusion that they were never designed to determine the effectiveness of immediate versus delayed hormonal therapy. Recently, Kozlowski et al. (1991) have reviewed the literature in favor of immediate hormone therapy. Randomized prospective trials are in process now to clarify this question, for example the European Organization for Research and Treatment of Cancer (EORTC) trial No. 30891 (Chairman U.E. Studer, Bern).

Another highly controversial topic is the form of androgen suppression (partial versus total androgen deprivation). For overview of current endocrine treatment and references regarding total androgen deprivation see Table 4. In general, protocols with total androgen deprivation have shown slightly better results with respect to objective response, delay in time to progression and survival. The benefits must always be weighed against quality of life and costs (Smith, 1991).

The role of chemotherapy in prostate cancer is not yet established. Less than 10 % of patients with hormone-refractory stage D2 disease treated with various chemotherapeutic agents experience complete or partial responses (Eisenberger, 1988). Moreover, the duration of such responses is short-lived and toxicity is considerably high. Commonly used single agents are Doxorubicin, Cyclophosphamide, Cisplatin, 5-Fluorouracil, Estracyt, Methotrexate and Hydroxyurea. Commonly used drug combinations are Cyclophosphamide plus Doxorubicin, Cisplatin plus Doxorubicin, Doxorubicin plus 5-Fluorouracil plus Mitomycin C, Cyclophosphamide plus Methotrexate plus 5-Fluorouracil and Cyclophosphamide plus Doxorubicin plus 5-Fluorouracil (Eisenberger, 1988).

Table 4. Current first-line endocrine treatment

- Androgen withdrawal
  - – Bilateral orchiectomy
  - – LH-RH agonists
    - Goserelin (Zoladex®)
    - Leuprolide (Lupron®)
    - Triptorelin (Decapeptyl®)
  - – Diethylstilbestrol
  - [– Estramustine phosphate (Estracyt®)]
- Androgen blockade
  - – Steroidal antiandrogens
    - Cyproterone acetate (Androcur®)
  - – Pure antiandrogens
    - Flutamide (Flucinom®)
    - Nilutamide (Anandron®)
- Total androgen deprivation (protocols)
  Combination of androgen withdrawal and androgen blockade
  - – Orchiectomy plus nilutamide (Beland et al., 1990; Janknegt et al., 1993)
  - – Leuprolide plus flutamide (Crawford et al., 1989)
  - – Leuprolide plus nilutamide (Labrie et al., 1983)
  - – Goserelin plus flutamide (Tyrrell et al., 1991)

Current efforts in the development of new systematic approaches for cancer in general focus on various biological response modifiers or other drugs that produce their cytotoxicity by inhibiting tumor growth factors mediated mechanisms. Suramin for example was able to induce objective responses in clinical trials, but only at the price of substantial toxicity (Linehan et al., 1990). In vitro tissue cultures have shown suramin to be cytostatic rather than cytocidal (Peehl et al., 1991). In light of the long doubling time of prostate cancer (see chapter 2.4.), cell cycle-nonspecific agents will be required in the future.

II. Natural history

2.1 Dilemma of latent prostate cancer

The natural history of prostate cancer has long been regarded as highly unpredictable. Whitmore's (1973) view of the natural course is depicted in Figure 5. The discrepancy between histologically identifiable (40 %) and clinically diagnosed (8 %) carcinomas (Stamey et al., 1993c) led to a considerable diagnostic and therapeutic dilemma. It has been asked enigmatically "Is cure necessary in whom it is possible, and is cure possible in whom it is necessary?" (Whitmore, 1988).

Rich (1935) first reported the dichotomy, observing that only one third of the patients with prostate cancer found at autopsy were recognized clinically as having the disease. His observations, however, were limited because he examined only one section of the prostate from each patient. In 1954, Franks in London systematically sectioned prostates transversely at 4 mm intervals in 220 patients who died of other diseases (Franks, 1954). Overall, in 38 % of cases he found unsuspected prostate cancer. These tumors were indistinguishable histologically from active clinical cancers; 75 % had infiltration of the capsule, 38 % had vascular invasion, 32 % had infiltration of nodules of benign prostatic hyperplasia and 6 % had invasion of the seminal vesicles. Since prostate cancer was responsible for only 1.4 % of all deaths in the United Kingdom in men over 50 years of age (Franks, 1956), he concluded that this type of tumor had the morphological and some of the biological characters of true malignancy, but lacked the capacity for rapid growth (Franks, 1954). The term "latent" carcinoma of the prostate prevailed for almost 40 years though no formal study has ever been able to sustain Franks' concept of latency.

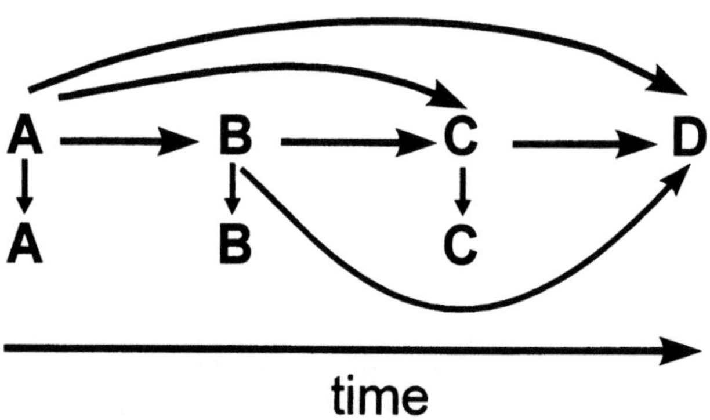

Fig. 5. Stage progression of prostatic cancer (from: Whitmore, 1973).

2.2 Concept of biologic tumor progression

Contemporarily with Franks, Leslie Foulds, another pathologist in London, developed his concept of biologic tumor progression (Foulds, 1954; Foulds, 1958). This concept is based on the assumption that the biologic aggressiveness of a tumor is correlated with the passage of time and with cumulative cell cycles. It includes that early (small) cancers can not metastasize, that mitosis in cancer cells generates heterogeneity and that the probability of metastasis increases with mass doublings, i.e. volume. Furthermore, it includes that higher grades (Gleason 4 and 5) evolve from better grades with the passage of time and that the percentage of grade 4+5 at any volume distinguishes faster from slower progression.

This volume-related concept has been validated in recent years by evidence from cell biology studies (Hanahan, 1989; Nicolson, 1987; Sager, 1989). Progression appears to be based on an inherent genetic instability in most types of malignant cells; they spontaneously accumulate mutational events on a random basis, with a cumulative probability that is proportional to the number of cell divisions the tumor has undergone (Cohen and Ellwein, 1990; Goldie, 1987; Goldie and Coldman, 1979). Because progression is probabilistic (Goldie, 1987), it carries an element of unpredictability for any cancer in any organ, for any cell in that cancer, and for any given mitosis of that cell. But probability is not selective, and it can not provide a basis for discriminating two biologic races within a single type of malignancy.

2.3 Tumor volume and Gleason grade

The important concept of biologic tumor progression has been confirmed by McNeal (1969) in his classic work on the origin and development of carcinoma in the prostate. On the basis of volume distribution data from 45 prostate cancers in 134 autopsies, McNeal proposed that there were not two types of prostate cancer (latent and clinically aggressive) but a single species having a slow growth rate with a biologic malignant potential that was closely linked to tumor size.

2.3.1 Determination of tumor volume

The original Stanford method for precise determination of tumor volume in prostate cancer has been described in great detail (Stamey et al., 1988): Immediately after radical prostatectomy, the seminal vesicles were first removed and incised in the coronal plane. Tissue was trimmed from the bladder neck and apical urethra for microscopic study of surgical margins. The external surface of the prostate was stained with indelible dye. After the specimen was weighed and measured, it was immersed in 37 % formalin overnight and serially blocked at 3 mm intervals with a specially constructed metal frame with a knife guide to ensure uniform thickness. Sections were taken transversely, perpendicular to the rectal surface, and they were displayed sequentially and identified with labels in reverse alphabetical order, beginning with Z at the prostatic apex. Between 9 and 12 levels usually were obtained, and each level was separated into right and left halves, for a total of 18 to 24 slides for the entire gland. All tissue sections were routinely processed into paraffin, and slides were cut at 7 μm from the rostral surface and stained with hematoxylin and eosin.

Cancer volume was determined from an ink tracing on each slide of the exact tumor outline as seen on microscopic inspection at low magnification (40x); questionable areas were confirmed at higher magnification. Sequential outline maps of the prostate and carcinoma were traced for each level of section through the gland at a magnification of 3x. With a Compaq computer with digitizing pad, the area of tumor at each level of section was determined. Volume was calculated as the sum of tumor areas at different levels multiplied by the section thickness (3 mm). This figure then was multiplied by a factor of 1.5 to correct for tissue shrinkage during processing, a factor determined by previous comparisons of the areas of fresh and processed tissue sections of prostates.

Pictorial reconstruction of the entire prostate together with its carcinoma was displayed as serial levels on a single sheet of paper by tracing at a magnification of 1 x (Figure 6). The map included outlines of benign prostatic hyperplasia nodules, extent of regions of complete tumor penetration of the capsule and any areas where tumor appeared to have been transected at operation. Capsule penetration by carcinoma was quantitated microscopically. The extent of complete penetration of each slide was indicated by an ink line drawn along the tissue border (Figure 6), and total extent of complete penetration was recorded as the sum of ink line lengths in millimeters.

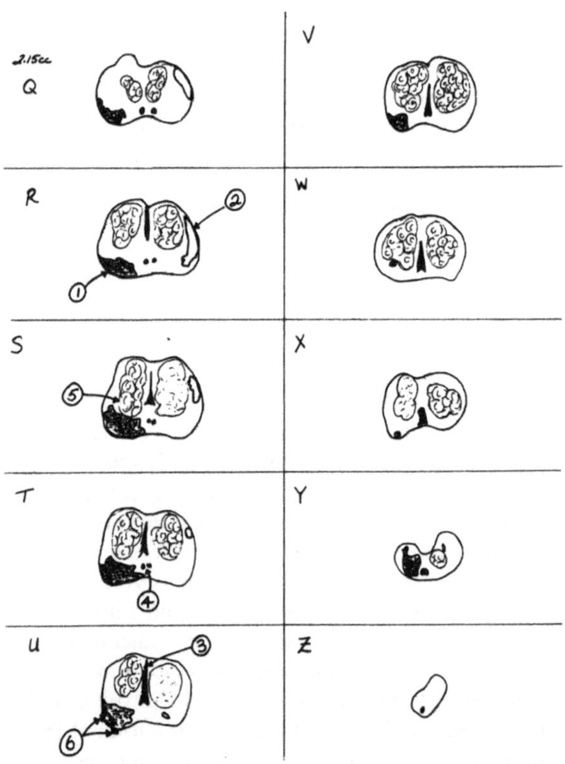

Fig. 6. Histological tracings of serially blocked 3 mm sections of prostate from apex (Z) to vesical neck (Q) in 68-year old man whose gland weighed 56 grams at radical prostatectomy. 1, primary cancer 2.2 cc in total volume in right lobe in all sections Z through Q. 2, second incidental primary cancer, volume 0.7 cc, in sections T to Q. 3, urethra. 4, ejaculatory ducts. 5, benign prostatic hyperplasia in sections Y through Q. 6, capsular penetration into periprostatic fat. These 2 areas extended 4 mm in total length (from: Stamey et al., 1988).

Seminal vesicle invasion and unsuspected, microscopic lymph node metastases were quantitated. The percentage of cancer invasion into each coronal section of seminal vesicle was estimated and recorded. For the right and left node dissections, the total number of nodes and the number involved by carcinomas were noted.

Carcinoma grade was determined by the Gleason system (Gleason, 1977; Gleason et al., 1974). Every histological pattern, grades 1 to 5, present in the carcinoma was recorded using all of the sections that contained tumor. An estimate was made of the percentage of the total cancer represented by each Gleason pattern seen.

2.3.2 Autopsy series

Further evidence that carcinoma seen at necropsy, clinically detected carcinoma, and metastatic disease represent different phases along the biological continuum of a single type of cancer was presented by McNeal and colleagues (1986). In 100 prostates with carcinoma taken at necropsy, tumor volume was related to differentiation and to the presence or absence of capsule invasion, seminal vesicle invasion, and metastasis as indices of aggressive behavior.

The volume distribution of the 100 tumors was such that the (microscopic) cancers with the smallest volume were the most numerous, with an exponentially declining frequency at successive increasing volumes (Figure 7). Eighty percent of the tumors were smaller

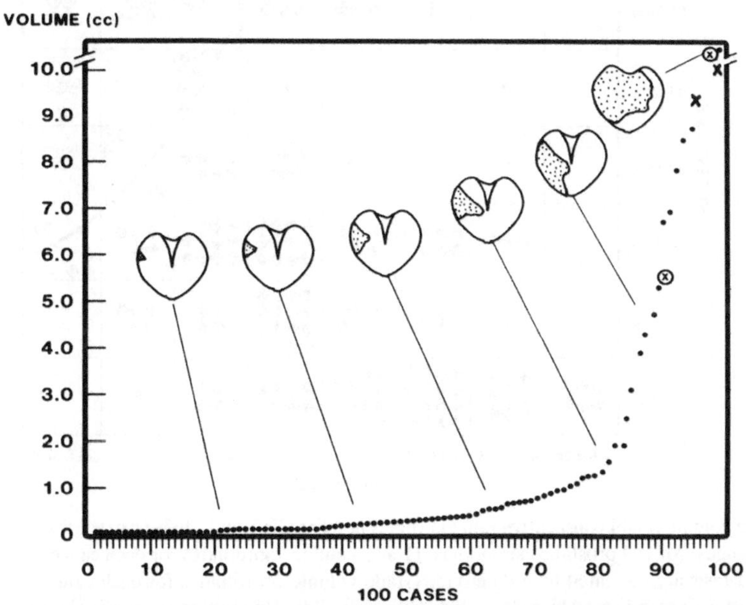

Fig. 7. Volume distribution of 100 prostate tumors in rank order. Inserts show approximate appearance at selected tumor volumes of coronal section through prostate. × distant metastases; ⊗ death from metastatic tumor (from: McNeal et al., 1986).

than 1.4 cc and 10 % were larger than 5.4 cc, including the four cases of distant metastases. Seven of the 100 tumors had seminal vesicle invasion, and the smallest of these measured 3.1 cc. The distribution of Gleason histological grades as a function of volume showed a prominent trend toward progressive loss of differentiation with increasing volume. None of the tumors larger than 0.17 cc was grade 1 or 2; by contrast, two of the metastatic carcinomas were grade 4 and two were grade 5. McNeal et al. (1986) concluded that these findings were consistent with their hypothesis of the coordinate evolution of morphologic and biologic malignant features in prostate cancer, at least in this selected group of autopsy carcinomas.

2.3.3 Radical prostatectomy series

The observations on the relationship of progression to volume and grade have been confirmed in the first 209 radical prostatectomies performed at Stanford University Medical Center (McNeal et al., 1990b). In 29 stage A cancers and 180 stage B cancers, tumor vol-

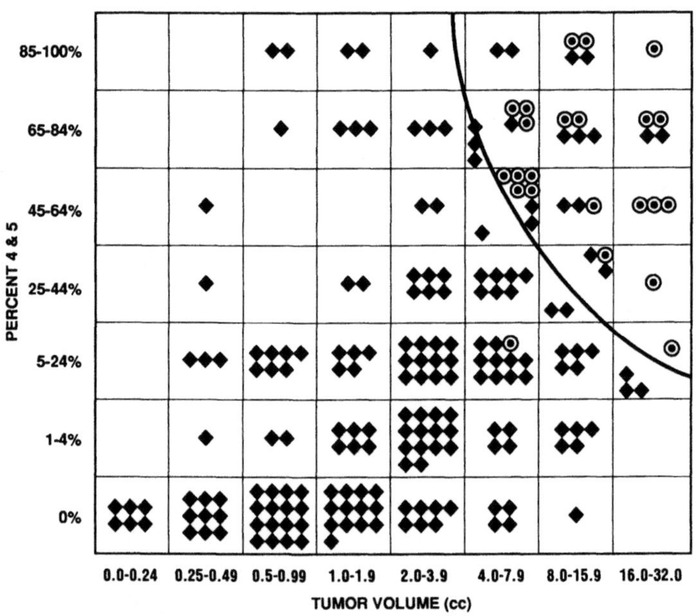

Fig. 8. Log volume (eight consecutive ranges) versus percent Gleason histologic pattern 4 – 5 cancer (consecutive ranges) for 209 prostatic carcinomas. Grade-volume coordinates for each cancer without lymph node metastasis are indicated by a diamond. Grade-volume coordinates for each cancer having lymph node metastasis are indicated by a clear circle with central dot. Those sets of coordinates that correspond to 3.2 cc of Gleason histologic pattern 4-5 cancer (cancer volume x percent of pattern 4 – 5) are joined by a curved line. There are 38 data points (cases) with more than 3.2 cc Gleason histologic pattern 4 – 5 cancer and 171 cases with less than 3.2 cc of pattern 4 – 5 cancer (from: McNeal et al., 1990b).

ume was determined according to the original Stanford method (chapter 2.3.1.) and Gleason histologic patterns of entire specimens were quantified. Generally, radical prostatectomy was not performed if pelvic lymph nodes with positive findings were demonstrated on frozen section. However, in 23 of 209 patients (11 %) lymph nodes were negative on frozen section but proved positive on permanent section.

If tumor volume as a single parameter was used to predict lymph node metastasis, none of the 125 patients (0 %) with volumes of less than 4 cc had positive nodes, whereas 23 of the 84 patients (27 %) with volumes of more than 4 cc were positive (Figure 8). The difference became even clearer, when tumor volume and histologic grade were combined. Only 1 of 171 patients (0.58 %) with less than 3.2 cc pure Gleason grade 4+5 had pelvic lymph node involvement compared to 22 of 38 patients (58 %) with more than 3.2 cc pure Gleason grade 4+5 (Figure 8). McNeal and coworkers (1990b) concluded that the absolute volume of the poorly differentiated portion of the cancer is most closely related to the biologic capacity for pelvic lymph node metastasis. Therefore, inaccuracy in clinical estimation of volume and grade rather than unpredictable biologic behavior are the main determinants of inadequate prediction for the individual patient.

Reports from other institutions have confirmed these findings. Lowe and Listrom (1988) analyzed stage A prostate cancer and showed convincingly that increasing grade and volume of the transurethrally resected tumor were highly related to progression. Schmassmann and Mihatsch (1983) demonstrated that the tumor size and the frequency of perineural space invasion increased with histologic dedifferentiation. Cumming et al. (1990) studied patients with carcinoma of the prostate who required two transurethral resections of the prostate, on average 2.4 years apart. They concluded that the natural history of prostate cancer, whether treated immediately or expectantly, was to dedifferentiate with time.

2.4 Growth pattern and doubling time*

Experimental studies have shown that prostate cancer has a slow growth rate when compared to other tumors (Meyer et al., 1982; Nemoto et al., 1989). On the basis of indirect evidence from volumes of incidental carcinomas in autopsy series (McNeal, 1969; McNeal et al., 1986) and unsuspected carcinomas in cystoprostatectomy specimens for bladder cancer (Stamey et al., 1993c), it has been proposed that prostate cancer follows a simple exponential growth curve with a constant long doubling time throughout its entire natural history. However, these determinations fail to reveal whether there is prognostic predictability in the histologic evolution of cancer with time. They are based on morphologic evaluation at a single point in time.

The estimation of approximate prostate cancer volume non-invasively in the individual patient with clinical carcinoma has become possible. A linear relationship has been demonstrated between serum PSA level and cancer volume. On average, a 3.5 ng/ml elevation of PSA reflects 1 cc (or 1 ml) of cancer, whether the cancer is within the prostate or extracapsular (Stamey et al., 1989; Stamey et al., 1987). In addition to these clinical inves-

* The Heinrich Warner Prize 1991/92 and Prize of the Swiss Institute for Applied Cancer Research (SIAK)/Essex 1993

tigations, animal studies have confirmed that the serum level of PSA is proportional to the volume of subcutaneously implanted, human prostate cancer (Csapo et al., 1988). The Yang polyclonal assay was used in these studies. Because serum PSA is proportional to prostate cancer volume, serial PSA determinations in the absence of any therapy to the prostate should reflect tumor growth rate and the shape of the growth curve.

2.4.1 Materials and methods

Forty-three patients with histologically proven prostate cancer who were referred to Stanford University Medical Center between February 1985 and April 1989 were followed up with serial serum PSA determinations. Only patients with two or more PSA determinations at least 12 months apart were included in this study. Between the initial and final PSA determinations, there was neither a specific treatment for prostate cancer (radical prostatectomy, radiation therapy, hormonal therapy, chemotherapy), nor any manipulation, e.g. transurethral resection or prostate biopsy.

The mean age of the patients at time of initital PSA determination was 71 years (range, 51 – 83 years). The mean follow-up from initial to final PSA determination was 30 months; the median follow-up was 26 months (range, 12 – 63 months).

The clinical stages at time of initial PSA determination are shown in Table 5. Ten patients had undergone transurethral resection of their prostates (TURP) for presumably

Table 5. All 43 patients stratified according to increasing group doubling times (in months) and clinical disease stages

	Group						
Disease stage	5 (stable)	4 (> 48 mo)	3 (24 – 48 mo)	2 (12 – 24 mo)	1 (< 12 mo)	Total in each clinical stage	Clinically organ-confined versus nonorgan-confined
Clinically organ-confined							
PSA-Ca		1				1	
TRUS-Ca	2	2		1		5	
A1	1	2	1	1		5	
A2		5				5	n = 28
B1	1	2	1			4	
B2		3	4			7	
B3	1					1	
Clinically nonorgan-confined							
C		4			1	5	
D1	1	1	1	3		6	n = 15
D2			1		3	4	
Total	**6**	**20**	**8**	**5**	**4**	**43**	

benign obstructive disease (five patients with stage A1; five with stage A2). Their initial PSA determination was obtained at least four weeks after TURP, when serum PSA had fallen to a steady state and falsely high initial PSA determination caused by the resection could be avoided. Twelve patients with clinical stage B cancers were substaged by the Stanford clinical classification (Stamey and Kabalin, 1989) (Figure 3). Five patients had clinical stage C disease, with palpable invasion of the seminal vesicles; six had stage D1 and four had metastatic stage D2 disease. Of the remainder, five patients had normal results at DRE but abnormal results of TRUS; biopsies were performed and showed prostate cancer (TRUS-Ca). Finally, one patient had normal results of DRE and TRUS, but had an elevated PSA, which led to a positive result on a transrectal, ultrasound-guided biopsy (PSA-Ca). For this analysis, we have considered clinical stages PSA-Ca, TRUS-Ca, A1, A2, B1, B2, and B3 to be clinically confined to the prostate (clinical stage B3 or less), and clinical stages C, D1, and D2 to be non-confined (clinical stage C or greater).

After the final PSA determination, 20 (47 %) patients received subsequent treatment: 9 (21 %) patients received hormonal therapy; 6 (14 %) underwent radical prostatectomy; and 5 (12 %) were treated with radiation therapy. Twenty-three (53 %) patients received no treatment. Of the six patients who had radical prostatectomy, the volume of their cancer and that of their benign prostatic hyperplasia (BPH) was measured by the Stanford technique (chapter 2.3.1.). The Gleason grade was determined for their entire cancer, based on 3 mm step sections.

Among the patients for whom treatment was delayed, eight refused therapy; ten were thought to have cancer too small to warrant treatment (most patients with clinical stage A disease); ten had no symptoms with advanced disease (clinical stages C, D1, and D2); nine were too old or in poor health; five had stable PSA levels and wanted to wait; and one insisted on a radical prostatectomy after being followed up for 24 months with only a microscopic focus of cancer.

For 22 patients, three or more PSA determinations obtained between the initial and final PSA determination were available, i.e. five or more values overall (mean, 6.8 determinations; range, 5 – 12 determinations). The distribution of clinical stages in these patients is similar to that of the 21 patients for whom we have only initial and final serum PSA determinations during the period of observation.

PSA was determined by the Yang assay, a polyclonal radioimmunoassay (Pros-check PSA, Yang Laboratories, Bellevue, WA). Intraassay and interassay coefficients of variation have been published (Stamey et al., 1987). All bloods was drawn on an ambulatory basis before rectal examination. PSA levels for a given point of time are highly reproducible. In a previous study we obtained two consecutive serum samples within 6 weeks from 31 ambulatory patients with newly diagnosed prostate cancer (Stamey et al., 1987). In the second sample, PSA had increased by 2 ± 22 %, which was not significant as indicated by the p values for any difference from a ratio of 1.00 for the two serum values. Thus, when connecting two PSA values from different points of time (in the current study at least 12 months apart), this line should be valid.

PSA doubling time (T') was calculated according to the formula

$$T' = \frac{\log 2 \text{ x } t}{\log(\text{final PSA}) - \log(\text{initial PSA})}$$

where t is the time from initial to final PSA determination in months.

Slides of the TURP chips or needle biopsy cores obtained at outside facilities were reviewed at Stanford. The Gleason grading system was used for histologic assessment. We report the sum of the primary and secondary Gleason grades (Gleason score).

2.4.2 Results

Growth Curve of Prostate Cancer

Twenty-two patients had a total of five or more PSA determinations during a period of more than 12 months. Ten of 12 patients whose cancer was clinically confined to the prostate at initial PSA determination are represented in Figure 9, top and bottom; only one of these patients had disease that advanced to nonorgan-confined status at final PSA determination. Nine of the ten patients who had nonorgan-confined disease at initial PSA determination are represented in Figure 10, top and bottom. For both subgroups, the intermediate PSA values closely followed a straight line connecting initial and final values on a log-PSA versus time scale (Figures 9 and 10). A linear relationship also was seen for the one patient with nonorgan-confined and two patients with organ-confined disease; data from these patients are not shown because the initial and final PSA determinations were stable (Figure 11, clinical stages D1, B1, and TRUS-Ca/B2).

Thus, the increase of serum PSA was judged to trace an exponential (log-linear) curve throughout the measured interval for all stages. On the basis of these findings, we included in our analysis 21 additional patients in whom only initial and final PSA determinations were known. Data of the entire group were evaluated in terms of a single number, the tumor doubling time.

Doubling Time, Stage, and Grade

Among the total of 43 patients, 37 (86 %) had an increase of PSA during the follow-up period, whereas six (14 %) had PSA levels that remained stable. This distribution is similar to the initial group of 22 patients for whom multiple PSA values were available.

Among the patients with stable disease (Figure 11), the final PSA determination averaged 92 % of the initial PSA determination, within the range of test accuracy on repeat determinations (Stamey et al., 1987). Local progression by digital rectal examination was undetectable in five of these six patients and may have been artifactual in the sixth patient (biopsy may have masked the nodule at initial examination). Bone scans remained consistently normal.

Doubling times varied from less than 12 months in four patients (Figure 12) to more than 24 months in most patients (Figure 13). Table 5 shows that in the category of clinically organ-confined disease, 26 of 28 patients (93 %) had a doubling time of more than 24 months; a doubling time of more than 24 months was found in 8 of 15 patients (53 %) with clinically nonorgan-confined disease. This difference was statistically significant using a chi-square test ($p = 0.01$).

It should be noted that seven of nine patients with doubling times of less than 24 months had clinically nonorgan-confined disease (Table 5). Among this group, all three patients who had distant metastases had doubling times of less than 12 months. Only one of four patients who had distant metastases (stage D2) had a doubling time of more than 24 months (Figure 13). Conversely, five of six patients with stable PSA values (Figure 11) and 15 of 20 with doubling times longer than 48 months had organ-confined disease (Figure 13). These two groups probably represent cancers of smaller volumes, as indicated in Table 6, by median initial PSA values of 5.7 and 10.7 ng/ml, respectively. By contrast, the initial median PSA value was 27.3 ng/ml in patients with doubling times of 12 – 24 months, and it was 26.9 ng/ml in those with doubling times of less than 12 months, consistent with much larger tumor volume.

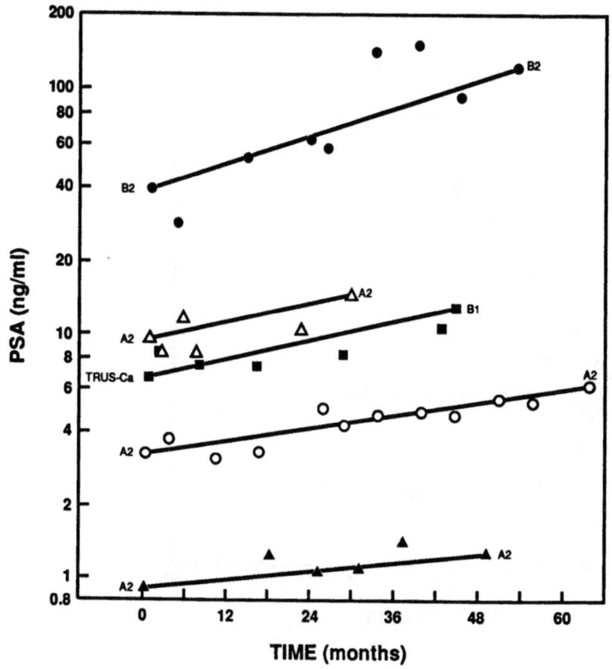

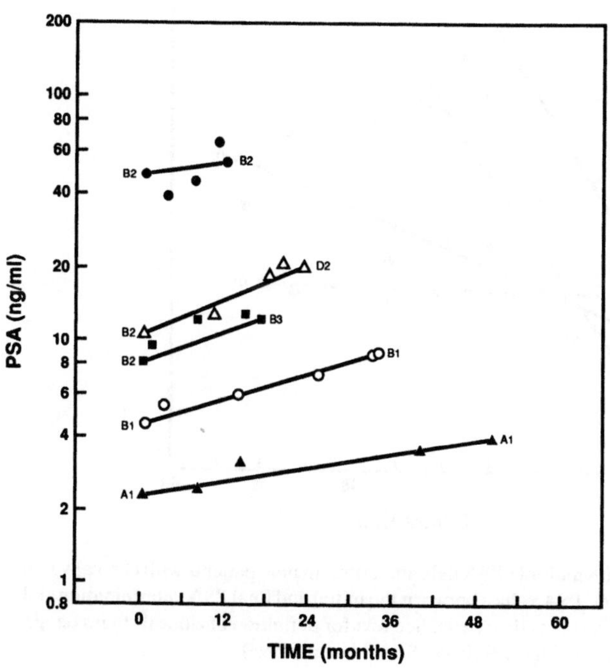

Fig. 9. Top and bottom. Follow-up with multiple PSA determinations in nine patients with clinically confined cancers (stages B3 and less) and one patient whose disease progressed from stage B2 to stage D2. PSA values between the initial and final PSA determinations follow the connecting line on the log-PSA versus time scale. See text for definition of clinical stages (stages PSA-Ca to D2). Symbols ●, ○, ▲, △, ■ used only to distinguish points of PSA for individual patients (from: Schmid et al., 1993).

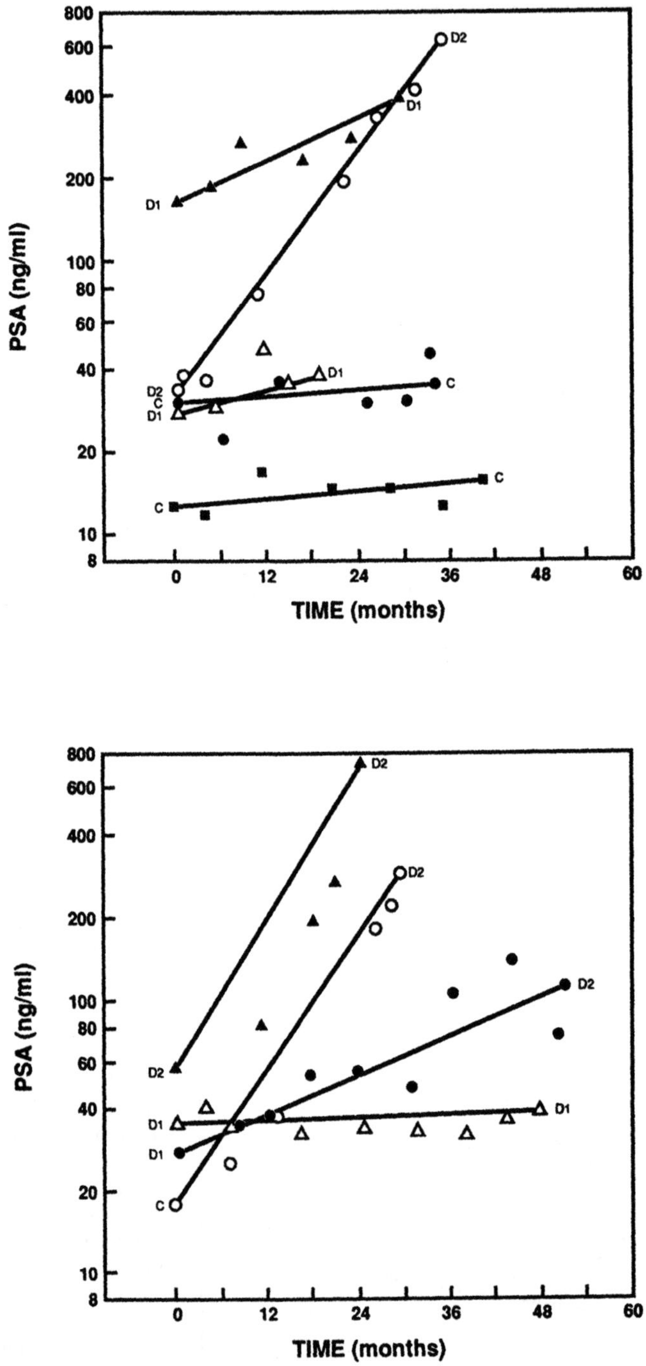

Fig. 10. Top and bottom. Follow-up with multiple PSA determinations in nine patients with clinically non-confined cancers (stages C and greater). PSA values between the initial and final PSA determinations follow the connecting line on the log-PSA versus time scale. See text for definition of clinical stages (stages PSA-CA to D2). Symbols same as those in Figure 9 (from: Schmid et al., 1993).

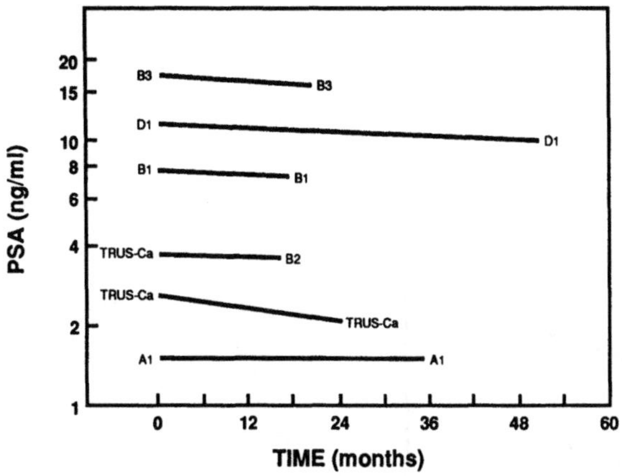

Fig. 11. Lines connect initial and final PSA determinations on a log-PSA versus time scale. Six patients with essentially stable PSA levels are represented. They had an average of 9 PSA determinations each (range, 4 – 15 determinations). See text for definition of clinical stages (stages PSA-Ca to D2) (from: Schmid et al., 1993).

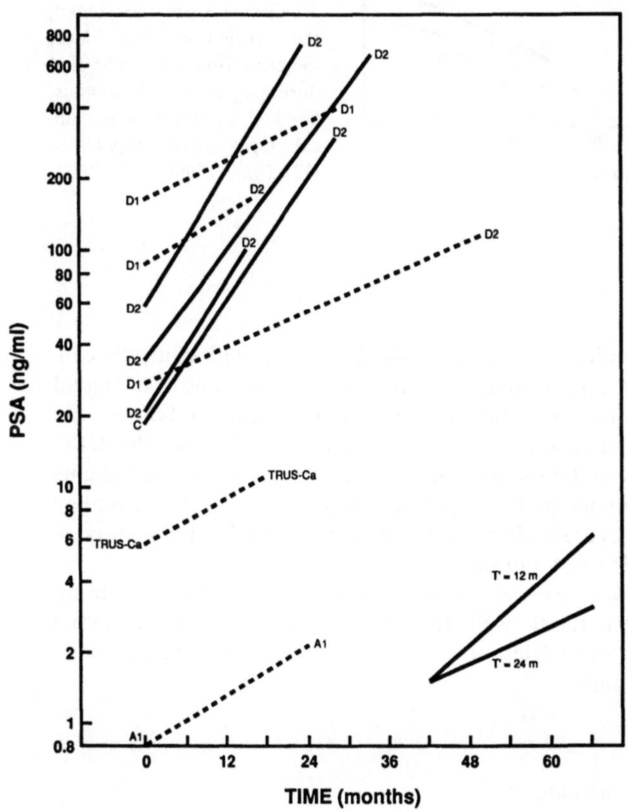

Fig. 12. Lines connect values of initial and final PSA determinations on a log-PSA versus time scale. Four patients (solid lines) with a doubling time (T') of less than 12 months and five patients (dashed lines) with T' of 12 – 24 months are represented. See text for definition of clinical stages (stages PSA-Ca to D2) (from: Schmid et al., 1993).

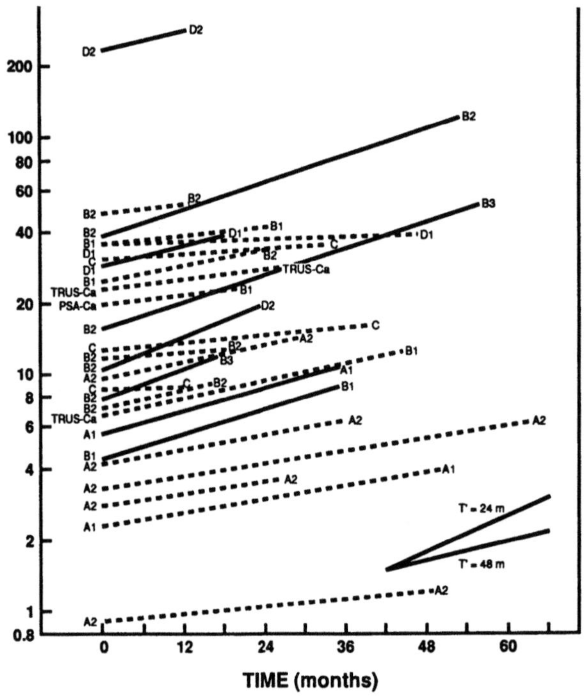

Fig. 13. Lines connect values of initial and final PSA determinations on a log-PSA versus time scale. Eight patients (solid lines) with doubling times (T') of 24 – 48 months and 19 patients (dashed lines) with T' longer than 48 months are represented. One patient in this group with clinical stage A1 disease is not represented; the patient's PSA level increased from 0.4 to 0.5 ng/ml during a period of 39 months. See text for definition of clinical stages (stages PSA-Ca to D2) (from: Schmid et al., 1993).

Data of the two groups are combined in Figure 14; the 27 patients with clinically con-ed cancer throughout the follow-up period had a median initial PSA value of 6.7 ng/ml d doubling time of 69.3 months. For the 15 patients with nonorgan-confined cancer, the dian initial PSA value was 30.8 ng/ml and median doubling time was 43.0 months. If the ubling times of the six patients who had stable PSA levels and those of the five patients ose increase in PSA was less than or equal to 1 ng/ml are excluded, the median doubling ne for organ-confined cancers decreases from 69 to 50 months and that for nonorgan-nfined cancers decreases from 43 to 24 months.

Higher histologic grades also were associated with faster doubling times (Table 6). ere was a statistically significant relationship ($p = 0.05$, using chi-square analysis) tween Gleason score 6 or lower versus Gleason score 7 or higher and a doubling time of ore versus one of less than 24 months.

fect of BPH on Doubling Time Calculation

'H is known to elevate serum PSA levels at an average of 0.3 ng/ml per cc (or gram) of 'H tissue (Stamey et al., 1987). Cancer elevates PSA, on average, 3.5 ng/ml per cc of

Table 6. Relationship of prostate-specific antigen level (PSA) doubling time with median PSA, median clinical disease stage, and median Gleason score

Group no.	Doubling time (mo)	No. of patients	Median initial PSA (ng/ml)	Median final PSA (ng/ml)	Median initial stage	Median final stage	Median Gleason score	No. of patients with Gleason score	
								≤6	≥7
1	<12	4	26.9	470.5	D2	D2	7.5	1	3
2	12–24	5	27.3	112.8	D1	D1	7.0	2	3
3	24–48	8	13.0	29.1	B2	B3	6.5	4	4
4	>48	20	10.7	13.5	A2/B1	B1	6.0	18	2
5	Stable	6	5.7	5.5	A1/B1	B1/B2	6.0	4	2
Total		**43**						**29**	**14**

cancer (Stamey et al., 1989). Thus, any given serum level is composed of PSA from normal prostatic tissue (as great as 2.5 ng/ml by the Yang assay), benign hyperplastic tissue, and cancerous tissue.

Thus, we cataloged the error in doubling time estimation introduced by BPH, using measurements on the six prostate specimens from patients who had radical prostatectomies after the follow-up period (Table 7). There were three patients with significant BPH, and their measured BPH volume were similar (7.9 – 10.2 cc). One patient had a cancer volume of 1.2 cc, and his tumor doubling time had been overestimated by 75 %

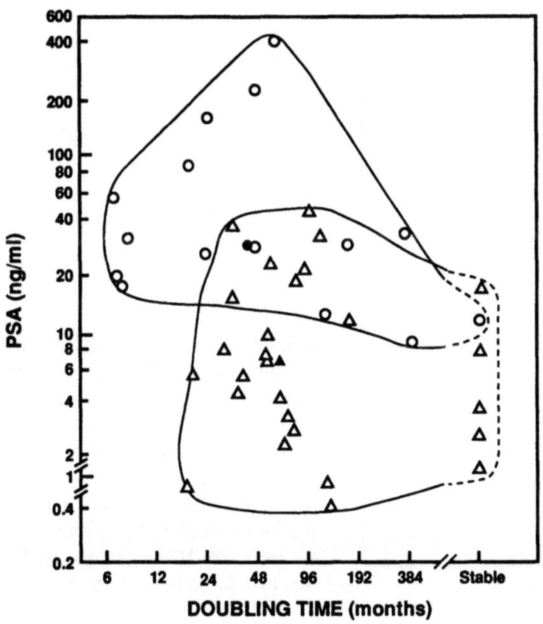

Fig. 14. Log (initial PSA level) versus log (PSA doubling time). △ 27 patients with clinically confined cancers throughout the follow-up period (excludes one patient whose tumor progressed from stage B2 to stage D2). ▲ median initial PSA value for this group was 6.7 ng/ml and median T' was 69 months. ○ 15 patients with nonorgan-confined cancers. ● median initial PSA value for this group was 30.8 ng/ml and median T' was 43 months (from: Schmid et al., 1993).

Table 7. Patients with subsequent radical prostatectomy

Patient no.	Clinical disease stage: Initial	Clinical disease stage: Final	Mo of follow-up in relation to initial and final PSA: Mo	Initial PSA (ng/ml)	Final PSA (ng/ml)	Cancer doubling time (mo): With BPH	Cancer doubling time (mo): Without BPH	Total weight of prostate (g)	Total cancer volume (cc)	Total BPH volume (cc)
1	A2	A2	26	2.8	3.6	71.7	71.7	20	3.65	0
2	B2	B3	17	7.9	11.9	28.8	28.8	22	5.30	0
3	PSA-Ca	B1	20	19.3	23.3	73.6	63.0	50	12.62	10.2
4	TRUS-Ca	B1	44	6.7	12.4	49.5	36.3	47	2.85	7.9
5	B1	B1	34	4.4	8.7	34.6	19.8	44	1.20	8.4
6	TRUS-Ca	TRUS-Ca	26	23.0	28.6	82.7	ND	183	0.01	ND

PSA: prostate-specific antigen; BPH: benign prostatic hyperplasia; ND: not determined

because of BPH before subtraction of PSA due to BPH. Similarly, a patient with cancer volume of 2.85 cc had overestimation of doubling time by 36 % before correction for BPH. In the other patient, who had 12.62 cc of cancer, tumor doubling time had been overestimated by 17 %.

It is clear that the presence of BPH contributes PSA to the serum in amounts that may produce erroneously long estimates of tumor doubling time. In Figure 15, the nature of the relationship is diagrammed. Increasing volume of cancer decreases the percent error with a tenfold steeper slope.

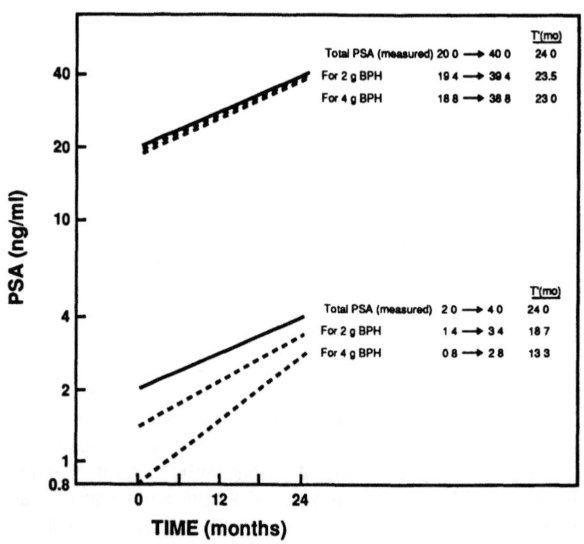

Fig. 15. Theoretical example for the influence of BPH and absolute PSA level on doubling times (T') of prostate cancer. Calculations are based on an average of 1 gram BPH equals 0.3 ng/ml PSA in the serum. The more BPH, the faster T', and the lower absolute PSA levels, the stronger the BPH influence on T'. See text for details (from: Schmid et al., 1993).

2.4.3 Discussion

When serum PSA was measured sequentially in patients with prostate cancer who received no treatment (Figures 9 and 10), there was an exponential (log-linear) increase in PSA with time in 86 % of the 43 patients we followed up, a linearity that allowed us to calculate a doubling time for PSA. Because the level of serum PSA is proportional to prostate cancer volume (Csapo et al., 1988; Stamey et al., 1989), we concluded that these exponential increases in PSA values are representative of tumor doubling times for prostate cancer volume. These observations have substantial consequences for the early diagnosis of prostate cancer in terms of annual screening with PSA.

The data in Tables 5 and 6 show that 79 % (34 of 43) of all the patients we have followed up without treatment have a tumor doubling time greater than 24 months; of the remaining 21 % whose cancers doubled in less than 24 months, seven of nine had advanced disease (clinical stages C, D1, and D2) when disease was first diagnosed. Sixty percent of our 43 patients had prostate cancers that required more than 48 months for the tumors to double in volume. Of most importance for therapeutic decisions, only 2 of 28 cancers thought to be clinically organ-confined (Table 5) doubled in less than 24 months, whereas 71 % doubled at rates exceeding 48 months.

The frequency of these surprisingly prolonged doubling times has not been previously recognized. When combined with our previous findings that malignant potential is strongly related to cancer volume (McNeal et al., 1986; McNeal et al., 1990b; Stamey et al., 1988), and that cancer volume can be estimated by serum PSA levels, this information has important clinical consequences. One consequence is the establishment of a firm scientific basis for deferring treatment in a select group of patients with prostate cancer whose tumor volume is estimated to be under a threshold level (Stamey et al., 1993c).

We have found that the probability of lymph node metastasis and extension of cancer locally beyond the prostate begins to increase above zero only in cancers larger than 4 cc (McNeal et al., 1990b). In the general population, approximately 80 % of all prostate cancers are less than 0.5 cc in volume (Stamey et al., 1993c), and most of these go undetected. In most patients, the current study indicates that it would require approximately 12 years (144 months) for a 0.5 cc cancer to reach 4 cc in volume if its doubling time was 4 years (48 months). However, rectal palpation and transrectal ultrasound are capable of detecting cancers as small as 0.2 cc (Stamey et al., 1993c; Stamey et al., 1988). Random sampling by needle biopsy and routine histologic examination of TURP chips can detect even smaller cancers. Thus, increasing interest in the screening of populations with no symptoms places at risk of diagnosis a large number of men in whom immediate treatment may be contraindicated. Criteria for distinction of this group have been lacking.

Doubling times of more than 48 months for 70 % of organ-confined cancers explains Whitmore's et al. (1991) observations regarding “expectant“ treatment of 29 patients with clinical stage B1 nodules, for which median follow-up of 10 years showed that all cancers had progressed, but they progressed so slowly that 15-year cancer-specific survival rates were 87 %. These values rival those of radical prostatectomy (Gibbons et al., 1984; Jewett, 1980) and radiation therapy of small cancers (Bagshaw et al., 1988). Because our morphometric studies indicate that 80 % of clinical stage B1 nodules range in volume from 0.2 to 4 cc (Stamey et al., 1988), the prolonged doubling times we have shown here suggest that the natural history of the untreated stage B1 nodule could be as long as 15 years before clinically detectable distant metastasis is present. Our doubling time data also are consistent with Scandinavian studies that suggest a long natural history without any treatment (Adolfsson and Carstensen, 1991; Johansson et al., 1992a).

Our observations that the relative amounts of BPH and prostate cancer could be measured in the six patients in this series who had radical prostatectomies (Table 7) led to the theoretical illustration in Figure 15. Assuming the average elevation of serum PSA caused by 1 cc of BPH to be 0.3 ng/ml (Perrin et al., 1991; Stamey et al., 1987), it is determined that the greater the amount of BPH that accompanies prostate cancer, the more likely the doubling time of the cancer will be overestimated. The less the amount of BPH, the more accurate the increase in serum PSA level will be in reflecting the doubling time of the cancer. As seen in Figure 15, this effect of BPH is critical primarily at lower PSA concentrations. The clinical importance of this observation is obvious. When following the doubling time of any prostate cancer by sequential measurements of serum PSA, the clinician should have an estimate of prostate size. The smaller the gland, the more accurately changes in PSA reflect the true doubling time of prostate cancer.

We have repeatedly emphasized the inaccuracy of DRE in estimating intracapsular cancer volume (Spigelman et al., 1986; Stamey et al., 1988). Although most stage B1 nodules are less than 4 cc in cancer volume, they range from 0.2 to 9 cc; stage B2 nodules (Figure 3) are 1 – 19 cc. DRE does not accurately reflect cancer volume in palpable stage B nodules, but the doubling time for prostate cancer shortens with increasing median initial and final stages (Table 6). Of six patients with pelvic lymph node metastases, there appeared to be a trend between tumor burden (number of positive nodes) and faster doubling times (data not shown).

Table 6 also demonstrates that an increasing Gleason biopsy score is associated with faster doubling times, despite the limitation imposed by TURP chips and needle biopsy cores representing only a fraction of the total cancer. The relationship between PSA doubling time (either more or less than 24 months) and Gleason score (6 or less or 7 or more) was significant by chi-square analysis at $p = 0.05$.

McNeal (1969) proposed that there were not two types of prostate cancer (latent and clinically aggressive) but a single species having a slow growth rate with a biologic malignant potential that was closely linked to tumor size. The information on slow doubling times for organ-confined cancer presented in this chapter appears to confirm that hypothesis. However, the data here show that doubling times gradually shorten with advancing clinical stage and that no slowing of tumor growth rates occurs in the advanced, metastatic D2 stage. Thus, there is no evidence of Gompertzian slowing of prostate cancer at the largest tumor burdens, which is said to be characteristic of other tumors (Shackney et al., 1978). It is possible that a few cancers may grow too slowly to measure an increase in size within these relatively short time spans. Indeed, in serial mammographic views of breast cancer shadows, Spratt et al. (1981) reported that 9 of 64 cancers (14 %) showed no growth.

We are concerned that the doubling time of serum PSA for patients with BPH in the absence of prostate cancer is unknown and could serve as an important control group for our 43 patients with prostate cancer who received no treatment. Carter et al. (1992b) have published a case-control study of serum PSA levels in men who were participants in a prospective aging study from the National Institute on Aging. Although the numbers of patients in the series are small, the group's PSA observations extended from 7 to 25 years before diagnosis. The rate of change in PSA levels distinguished patients with prostate cancer ($n = 18$) from patients with BPH ($n = 20$) and control subjects ($n = 16$) with a specificity of 90 % and 100 %, respectively. These observations appear to add validity to the data published here that a log-linear but slow increase in serum PSA is characteristic of prostate cancer and that "contamination" with BPH should be a minor problem.

However, we recognize that large BPH prostate glands can be associated with substantial increases in PSA levels (0.29 ± 0.09 ng/ml per cc of BPH tissue) (Stamey et al., 1987).

In these patients, it is unlikely that doubling time for PSA levels is as long as the 10-year period suggested by Carter et al. (1992b), and there is no evidence in our patients with clinical stage B who have received no treatment to support the observations by Carter et al. (1992b) that serum PSA levels increase as slowly as 0.75 ng/ml/year.

The problems with distinguishing cancer from BPH by a serial increase in PSA levels are additionally compounded by our recent observations on large, organ-confined, impalpable transition zone (BPH) prostate cancers, which are so anteriorly located that routine transrectal biopsies usually yield negative results (Stamey et al., 1993a). Longitudinal studies of 10 – 15 years on serum PSA levels in patients with BPH and no cancer clearly would be useful. Until such studies are available, the clinician must rely on our earlier observations, that, gram for gram, prostate cancer elevates serum PSA on average at least ten times as much as BPH (Stamey et al., 1987), and also on the data in this chapter that in the presence of untreated prostate cancer, PSA levels display a steady log-linear increase with the passage of time.

2.5 Impact on early diagnosis and management*

Based on prostate cancer incidence rates for the period 1973 – 1977 from the Surveillance, Epidemiology, and End Results (1981) Program of the National Cancer Institute and American total mortality rates for the year 1986 (National Center for Health Statistics, 1986), we calculated the probability at birth of a man having a diagnosis of prostate cancer made within his life to be 8.8 % (Stamey et al., 1993c). We then subtracted the incidence of microscopic stage A cancers too small to ever be clinically significant, which gave a final probability of 8 %. In chapter 2.3. strong evidence has been presented that the biologic aggressiveness (progression) of prostate cancer is a direct function of tumor volume. Therefore, we asked the question: what is the volume of the 8 % clinically significant prostate cancers in the general population? Stated another way, is there a threshold volume below which cancers are too small to ever become clinically significant in view of the long doubling time of prostate cancer (chapter 2.4.)?

We evaluated 139 consecutive, unselected patients who underwent radical cystoprostatectomy for bladder cancer at Stanford University Medical Center (Stamey et al., 1993c). Preoperatively none of these men had any evidence for simultaneously identifiable prostate cancer. At least two DRE were performed on each patient, 76 of these 139 patients had ambulatory PSA determinations (Yang polyclonal assay) and 51 had TRUS of their prostates prior to surgery. The cystoprostatectomy specimens underwent a detailed morphologic evaluation. The entire prostate was cut in 3 mm step sections according to the original Stanford method (chapter 2.3.1.) and tumor volume of every identifiable prostate cancer was exactly calculated.

In the 139 cystoprostatectomies for bladder cancer, 55 unsuspected prostatic carcinomas (40 %) could be identified, an incidence similar to previously reported unselected autopsy (Franks, 1954) and cystoprostatectomy specimen series (Montie et al., 1989). The age distribution of these 55 patients with prostate cancer was identical to the entire group of 139 men (median age, 65 years; range, 31 – 84 years), pointing out that it was an unselected

* Prize for Medicine 1992/93 and Prize of the Swiss Urological Association 1993

cohort. The volume distribution of the 55 unsuspected prostate cancers is shown in Figure 16. Two of the cancers were more than 1.5 cc in volume (1.4 % of the 139 patients), 6 were more than 1.0 cc (4.3 % of all patients), and 11 were more than 0.5 cc (7.9 %). Of the 76 cystoprostatectomy specimens from patients for whom we had serum PSA determinations, 32 (42 %) had prostate cancer, and 44 (58 %) did not. The level of PSA ranged from 0.3 – 21.1 ng/ml. The median PSA value in patients with prostate cancer was 2.5 ng/ml; it was 1.6 ng/ml in those patients without prostate cancer.

The tumor volume distribution of 55 unsuspected prostate cancers found incidentally at cystoprostatectomy for bladder cancer is exponential (Figure 16). Forty-four of these 55 prostatic carcinomas (80 %) were smaller than 0.5 cc; this pattern of distribution is in keeping with a previous autopsy series (McNeal et al., 1986). The other 11 prostate cancers of more than 0.5 cc represent 7.9 % of the total 139 patients and correspond to the 8 % risk for a man being diagnosed within his lifetime with a clinically significant tumor (Stamey et al., 1993c). Thus, a majority of carcinomas (80 %) has such a low tumor volume (less than 0.5 cc) that they will never get clinical significance in view of their long median doubling time of four years. This outcome has substantial consequences for early detection.

Primary diagnosis of prostate cancer is based on PSA and DRE with the serum marker as sole parameter being superior to rectal palpation (Catalona et al., 1991). While generally everybody agrees that a palpable nodule should be biopsied, the situation with a negative DRE – depending on serum PSA level – is controversial. Cooner and associates (1990) were able to demonstrate that with a negative palpation and a PSA of 4.1 – 10.0 ng/ml (Hybritech assay) 18 men had to undergo transrectal ultrasonography and six had to be biopsied to detect one carcinoma. For PSA values up to 4.0 ng/ml the corresponding numbers were 41 and nine. Hammerer and Huland (1991) found similar results in their series of 712 patients who underwent random-systematic biopsies. This low gain does not justify the considerable costs and expense of TRUS guided biopsies. Since in men with a PSA less than 10 ng/ml an incidentally present carcinoma would have a low tumor volume (Stamey

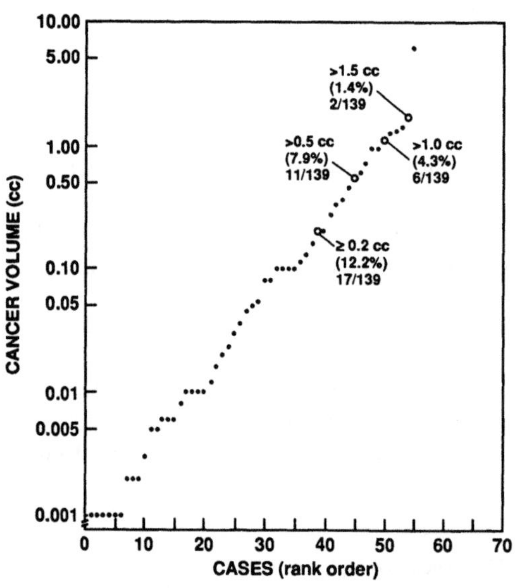

Fig. 16. Volume distribution of 55 unsuspected largest prostate cancers in 139 cystoprostatectomies. See text for details (from: Stamey et al., 1993c).

Table 8. Algorithm for early detection of prostate cancer

PSA (ng/ml) Yang assay (Hybritech assay)	DRE positive	negative
0.0–7.3 (0.0–4.0)	a	c
7.4–18.4 (4.1–10.0)	a	c
> 18.4 (> 10.0)	a	b

a TRUS guided biopsies; b TRUS guided systematic biopsies (Hodge et al. 1989b); c Follow-up (PSA and DRE)

et al., 1989) and since the doubling time is very long (chapter 2.4.), we suggest to follow these men annually with PSA and DRE (Schmid et al., 1994) (Table 8).

In the clinical Stanford series of more than 700 radical prostatectomies, patients with a tumor volume up to 4 cc – and perhaps even up to 6 cc – were cured almost without exception, if positive surgical margins could be avoided. A standardized method for accurate tumor volume estimation in radical prostatectomy specimens has been introduced and is presented in chapter 4.1. Limitations in the accurate estimation of cancer volume preoperatively reduce the practical value of the above findings. However, Hodge et al. (1989b) have shown an increase in accuracy of volume estimation by combining information from TRUS and six systematically placed needle biopsies. By measuring the percent of each biopsy occupied by cancer and the percent of Gleason grade 4 or 5 cancer on each biopsy and combining these data with serum PSA determination and ultrasound estimated volume, they have developed an algorithm that appears to provide sufficiently increased accuracy of volume estimation for clinical decisions. Therefore, we think we can practically estimate a volume threshold of 0.5 cc, below which treatment should not be considered, except in the young patient, and even in that instance treatment may be delayed for years.

The data presented here clearly demonstrate that in prostate cancer the goal is not to diagnose more and more insignificant tumors from the pool of carcinomas below 0.5 cc. Early diagnosis in prostate cancer is something unique and means diagnosis within the therapeutic window of 0.5 – 6 cc. In view of the extraordinary slow growth rate the time frame for appropriate diagnosis is about 10 years.

III. Selection criteria for radical prostatectomy

The surgical management of localized prostate cancer depends on patient selection. The appropriate candidate for radical prostatectomy should have disease that is confined to the prostate, an expected longevity that is longer than the natural history of his cancer, and no significant surgical risk factors.

The problem with clinical staging of prostatic carcinoma is predominantly understaging of disease (Catalona and Dresner, 1985; Elder et al., 1982; Stamey and McNeal, 1992). Unfavorable outcome has been reported for those patients with pathologically confirmed extraprostatic disease (Elder et al., 1982; Partin et al., 1993). More extensive surgery for locally advanced tumors does not improve results. Cystoprostatectomy and pelvic exenteration does not appear to be a curative endeavor and may be accompanied by significant morbidity (McCullough and Leadbetter, 1972; Moul and Paulson, 1991). Only 10 % or less of patients with clinical stage T3 tumors will be overstaged, that is, will actually have organ-confined disease (Bosch et al., 1987; Lange and Narayan, 1983).

Recently, the necessity of pelvic staging-lymphadenectomy prior to radical prostatectomy has been questioned by several investigators. Although it is true that a pelvic lymph node dissection can provide staging information that can be obtained by no other method, the procedure increases operating room time and can increase patient morbidity. Potential complications of bleeding, lymphocele, vascular and neurologic problems and infection occur in approximately 20 % of patients who undergo pelvic lymphadenectomy alone, regardless of how it is performed (Donohue et al., 1990; Kavoussi et al., 1993). Furthermore, this procedure is only diagnostic but not therapeutic (Gervasi et al., 1989). There might be subpopulations of patients in whom staging-lymphadenectomy can be omitted.

The objective of chapter III is to define clinical (preoperative) selection criteria which can reliably predict pathological outcome, i.e. which can separate organ-confined from nonorgan-confined prostate cancer.

3.1 Materials and methods

From February 1976 to June 1990 144 patients with adenocarcinoma of the prostate underwent bilateral pelvic lymphadenectomy and radical retropubic prostatectomy at our institution. Four patients were excluded from analysis: three had metastatic disease (M1) at time of radical prostatectomy and one had a false-positive fine needle aspiration (FNA) with no cancer present in the radical prostatectomy specimen (pT0). Of the remaining 140 patients (100 %) the mean age at time of surgery was 63.8 years, the median age was 65 years and the range was 45 to 76 years.

Tumors were classified according to the TNM-system from 1987 (see Table 1). There were 11 clinical stage T1 cancers (8 %), 108 clinical stage T2 cancers (77 %) and 21 clinical

Table 9. Clinical staging compared to pathological staging

		Pathological stage				
		pT1	pT2	pT3	pT4	
Clinical stage	T1	7	0	4	0	11
	T2	0	35	72	1	108
	T3	0	3	18	0	21
		7	38	94	1	140

stage T3 cancers (15 %) (Table 9). All 140 patients were clinically judged N0 M0. Staging was based on digital rectal examination (DRE) by at least two clinicians, chest X-rays and radioisotopic bone scans (BS). Additionally, from 1976 to 1980, vesiculography, bipedal lymphangiography and bone marrow biopsy of the pelvis were performed to rule out extraprostatic disease. These invasive procedures were replaced in 1980 by CAT scan of the pelvis and abdomen. From May 1987 to June 1989 magnetic resonance imaging (MRI) of the prostate with surface coils and transrectal probes, respectively was done. However, these investigations were performed for study purposes (Hering and Mueller, 1991) and did not influence selection for radical prostatectomy.

Diagnosis of prostatic carcinoma and preoperative grading was established by transurethral resection of the prostate (TURP) in 13 cases (9 %), by FNA in 62 cases (44 %), by biopsy in 61 cases (44 %) and in four cases (3 %) the method of grading was unknown. FNA was done fingerguided by the transrectal approach according to Franzen et al. (1960), yielding a cytologic diagnosis. For histology, either perineal or transrectal biopsies were performed. Transrectal ultrasound (TRUS) guided biopsies were introduced at our institution in 1989. The Dhom system was used for histologic or cytologic grading (Dhom, 1977; Mueller et al., 1980). Preoperatively, there were 30 G1 cancers (21 %), 68 G2 cancers (49 %) and 14 G3 cancers (10 %) (Table 10). For 10 cancers (7 %) no conclusive grade could be assigned (GX) and in another 14 cases (10 %) the first diagnostic attempt was false-negative. Finally, in four cases (3 %) the method of grading was unknown and these cases were excluded from this type of analysis.

For determination of serum markers all blood was drawn on an ambulatory basis prior to DRE and prior to any hormonal manipulation, i.e. in the untreated patient. Prostatic acid phosphatase (PAP) was measured with an enzymatic assay using thymolphthalein monophosphate as substrate (Roy et al., 1971) until 1983. This method was then replaced by the more sensitive radioimmunoassay (Huber et al., 1982). The upper limit for PAP at our institution for men with normal prostates or benign prostatic hyperplasia (BPH) was 3.1 ng/ml. Prostate-specific antigen (PSA) was first introduced in Switzerland by Huber and colleagues (1986). Starting with PSA determinations in November 1985 we used polyclonal radioimmunoassay test kits obtained from Yang Laboratories (Pros-check PSA, Bellevue, WA) and distributed in Switzerland by Travenol (Dietlikon, ZH). We defined an upper limit of 12 ng/ml for normal prostates and BPH.

In December 1987 autologous blood transfusion was instituted. Patients donated 2 – 4 units prior to their operation. From May 1989 patients received the pure antiandrogen flutamide (3 x 250 mg/day) in the two to three months before radical prostatectomy for downsizing of the prostate.

Table 10. Preoperative grade vs. definite grade

			Radical prostatectomy specimen				
			G1	G2	G3	GX	
Preoperative grading	G1	TURP	3	3	0	0	30
		FNA	1	2	2	0	
		Biopsy	2	8	8	1	
	G2	TURP	0	4	1	0	68
		FNA	0	16	19	0	
		Biopsy	0	16	12	0	
	G3	TURP	0	0	1	0	14
		FNA	0	0	5	0	
		Biopsy	0	0	8	0	
	GX	TURP	0	0	0	0	10
		FNA	0	3	3	0	
		Biopsy	1	2	1	0	
		TURP	0	1	0	0	14
	negative**	FNA	0	6	5	0	
		Biopsy	0	1	1	0	
			7	62	66	1	136*

* method of grading unknown in 4 cases; ** primary attempt false negative

Postoperatively, patients with pathologically confirmed capsular penetration or seminal vesicle invasion (pT3) and patients with pN1 lymph node status received adjuvant irradiation to the prostatic bed and to the pelvic lymph nodes. External beam radiotherapy was administered with 45 MV photons. A dose of 6000 cGy was delivered to the prostate and 4500 cGy to the pelvic lymph nodes calculated at the 85 % isodose contour. Patients were treated 5 days per week with 200 cGy per fraction. In general, this adjuvant treatment was initiated two months after radical prostatectomy.

3.2 Results

3.2.1 Clinical features

The relationship of clinical staging to final outcome is shown in Table 9. Overall, of 140 cases, pathological stage was correctly predicted in 60 cases (43 %). For clinical stages T1-2 there was a considerable error toward understaging. Of 119 clinically organ confined tumors, only 42 (35 %) were actually pT1-2. In clinical stage T3, 3 of 21 tumors (14 %) were overstaged.

In this series 49 of 140 patients (35 %) had positive pelvic lymph nodes on permanent sections (pN1-2). There was a higher probability for lymph node metastases with increasing clinical stages. Two of 11 stage T1 tumors (18 %) had positive nodes as compared to 33 of 108 stage T2 (31 %) and 14 of 21 stage T3 (67 %). In 38 cases the side of the palpable nodule (in clinical stages T2-3) and the side of lymph node metastases were both documented (Table 11). Preoperatively, in 19 of 38 cases (50 %) was the side of lymph node involvement correctly predicted by DRE.

The histological grade of TURP-chips corresponded in 8 of 13 cases (62 %) to the final grade in the radical prostatectomy specimen (Table 10). Four cases were undergraded; there was no overgrading and one of 13 cases (8 %) was false-negative. For FNA, cytological grading corresponded to histology of the entire specimen in 22 of 62 tumors (35 %). Not a single tumor was overgraded, and 11 of 62 tumors (18 %) were missed at first attempt. Correct final grade was predicted by biopsy in 26 of 61 cancers (43 %). Again there was no overgrading, and 2 of 61 cases (3 %) were false-negative. Overall, for the three different grading modalities, preoperative tumor grading was in agreement with postoperative grading of the entire specimen in 56 of 136 cases (41 %) (Table 10).

3.2.2 Serum markers

Forty-four patients had determination of serum PSA prior to radical prostatectomy and 130 patients had PAP measurement. The values in relationship to pathological outcome are shown in Table 12. All mean and median values for PSA were above the normal cut-off level of 12 ng/ml for men with normal prostates or BPH, whereas all mean and median values for PAP were well within the normal range of up to 3.1 ng/ml. In 17 patients PSA was more than 30 ng/ml and only one patient (6 %) with PSA in that range had pathologically organ-confined cancer. PAP was 2.5 ng/ml or more in 17 patients and one patient (6 %) had pT1-2 pN0 status.

The relationship of cut-off levels for PSA and PAP to pathological status is depicted in Table 13. Seven of 13 pathologically organ-confined cancers (54 %) had an elevated (above normal) PSA value and 25 of 31 nonorgan-confined cancers (81 %) had an elevated PSA. In cases with positive lymph nodes, 10 of 11 (91 %) had above normal PSA values. The corresponding numbers for PAP were lower: none of the 38 pathologically organ-confined cancers (0 %) could be detected by an elevated PAP and only 9 of 92 nonorgan-confined cancers (10 %) had an elevated PAP. In cases with positive lymph nodes, 8 of 46 (17 %) had above normal PAP values.

Table 11. Side of the palpable nodule in clinical stages T2 – 3 compared to side of lymph node involvement

		Positive lymph nodes (pN1 – 2)			
		right	left	bilateral	
Clinical stages (T2 – 3)	right	6	4	2	12
	left	3	7	5	15
	bilaterial	2	3	6	11
		11	14	13	38

Table 12. Serum levels of PSA and PAP compared to pathological status

		organ-confined (pT1–2 pN0) n = 13	nonorgan-confined (pT1–4 pN0–2) n = 31	LN positive (pN1–2) n = 11
PSA (ng/ml)	mean	16.9	31.6	43.5
	median	13.1	30.8	50.0
	range	3.0–50.0	3.6–72.0	8.0–72.0
		organ-confined (pT1–2 pN0) n = 38	nonorgan-confined (pT1–4 pN0–2) n = 92	LN positive (pN1–2) n = 46
PAP (ng/ml)	mean	0.9	1.9	2.4
	median	0.9	1.0	1.0
	range	0.0–2.8	0.0–26.0	0.0–26.0

Forty patients had both, PSA and PAP, determinations prior to surgery. The two serum markers were in the normal range of less than 12 ng/ml and less than 3.1 ng/ml, respectively in 11 patients (27 %). PSA was elevated and PAP was normal in 25 of 40 patients (63 %); on the other hand, not a single patient had a normal PSA and an elevated PAP (0 %). Finally, both markers were above the normal values in 4 of 40 patients (10 %).

Additional serum parameters (hemoglobin, erythrocyte sedimentation rate, creatinine, alkaline phosphatase) were not considered for analysis. They are of certain significance only in metastatic prostate cancer (de Voogt et al., 1989; Johansson et al., 1992b). In this series of locally confined tumors, those parameters were in the normal range for all patients, as was performance status; thus patients were eligible for major surgery.

Table 13. Cut-off levels for PSA and PAP compared to pathological status

		organ-confined (pT1–2 pN0) n = 13	nonorgan-confined (pT1–4 pN0–2) n = 31	LN positive (pN1–2) n = 11
PSA (ng/ml)	<12	6	6	1
	≥ 12	7	25	10
		organ-confined (pT1–2 pN0) n = 38	nonorgan-confined (pT1–4 pN0–2) n = 92	LN positive (pN1–2) n = 46
PAP (ng/ml)	<3.1	38	83	38
	≥ 3.1	0	9	8

3.2.3 Radiological examinations

The results of radiological examinations have to be interpreted with caution since we do not know how many patients were precluded from radical prostatectomy based on positive CAT scans, vesiculograms and lymphangiograms. However, from personal experience with CAT scans I believe there were but a few patients with clearly documented extraprostatic disease in the pelvis and appearance of grossly involved lymph nodes, respectively.

Vesiculography was performed in 17 patients and was considered suspicious in two (one patient had pathologically documented seminal vesicle invasion, one did not). Of the other 15 patients with negative vesiculograms, four were false-negative (27 %). Bipedal lymphangiography was done in 27 patients. Three patients had suspicious findings and one proved to be pN0, one was actually pN1, and one was pN2. Of the 24 patients with negative lymphangiograms, five were false-negative (21 %).

The results of MRI investigations with surface coils and transrectal probes were published elsewhere (Hering and Mueller, 1991).

3.3 Discussion

Appropriate selection for radical prostatectomy is one of the major goals in clinically organ-confined carcinoma of the prostate. The ideal candidate for curative surgery would be the one in whom total extirpation of the cancer could be reliably predicted by preoperative parameters. Unfortunately, with current staging methods this is not the case and up to 60 % of patients actually have pathologically confirmed extraprostatic disease (Catalona and Dresner, 1985; Elder et al., 1982; Stamey and McNeal, 1992).

In our series of 140 consecutive radical prostatectomies we were in keeping with the literature with respect to the considerable extent of clinical understaging of prostate cancer. Pathological stage was in agreement with preoperative, clinical stage in only 43 % of cases (Table 9). We found a slightly higher proportion of clinical stage T3 cancers that were overstaged (14 %) when compared to the series of Bosch et al. (1987) and Lange and Narayan (1983), respectively. While DRE has been recognized as insufficient staging tool (Stamey and McNeal, 1992), hopes for more accurate prediction of organ-confined disease have been evoked through the introduction of PSA. In this series, mean and median PSA levels were increasing with advancing pathological status but there was a considerable broad range of values in the individual case (Table 12). However, it must be noted that only 6 % of patients with a PSA of more than 30 ng/ml had pathologically organ-confined tumor. Palken et al. (1990) found that PSA levels of more than 50 ng/ml (Hybritech assay) were strongly suggestive for pathological stage C and D disease. In the series of Sassine and Schulman (1993), all patients with PSA over 20 ng/ml (Hybritech assay) had extraprostatic tumor extension. As seen from Table 13, PSA is superior to PAP for each pathological category when cut-off values are used as a reference. Moreover, in the 40 patients in whom both serum markers were concomitantly determined, we did not find a single case with a normal PSA and an elevated PAP. Thus, in the presence of PSA, PAP does not yield any additional information. Stamey and coworkers (1987) were the first to convincingly documente the superiority of PSA over PAP. Wirth and Frohmueller (1992) could show that in all tumor stages, PSA was superior to PAP in detecting cancer of the prostate.

Since understaging is such a problem, neoadjuvant hormonal treatment has been tried in order to possibly downstage the tumor prior to radical prostatectomy. This theory of a combination of hormonal therapy and surgery was initially proposed by Scott and Boyd (1969). While there is no doubt that antiandrogen treatment can significantly lower serum PSA levels and shrink total prostatic volume (Kennedy et al., 1992; Oesterling et al., 1993), no consistant change in histological Gleason score was noted (Kennedy et al., 1992). Furthermore, in a retrospective pair-matched analysis, Oesterling and colleagues (1993) did not find any impact of preoperative androgen deprivation on maximal tumor dimension and pathological stage. In addition, hormonal pretreatment does not even appear to facilitate the surgical procedure (Macfarlane et al., 1993). From the fact that hormones are not cytotoxic and that hormone-resistant clones of cells are not effected, it is clear that clinical downsizing does not equate with pathologic downstaging. Based on these findings, we included patients who were pretreated with the non-steroidal antiandrogen flutamide for analysis.

Postoperatively, patients with pathologically established capsular penetration or seminal vesicle invasion (pT3) and patients with pN1 lymph node metastases received external beam radiation therapy. The role of this adjuvant treatment is not yet well defined. Kaplan and Bagshaw (1992) have reviewed results of post-radical prostatectomy radiotherapy from several studies. While patients with undetected microscopic metastases at time of radical prostatectomy will certainly not benefit from adjuvant radiotherapy, in cases of isolated local persistance or recurrence of tumor it is possible that irradiation may sterilize the local lesion and render the patient free of tumor. Lange and associates (1990) reported that after radical prostatectomy persistant local-regional disease was the predominant and possibly only residual disease in some patients who ultimately fail. These data are in keeping with the observations by Link et al. (1991) on two groups of patients with detectable PSA following radical prostatectomy. The first group had a persistant or immediately increasing PSA after surgery and adjuvant external beam radiation therapy was of limited value. In the second group, PSA showed a delayed increase and adjuvant therapy was more encouraging. Overall, adjuvant irradiation for pathological stage C seems to prolong disease-free survival (Stein et al., 1992) but does not affect ultimate survival (Eisbruch et al., 1994; Paulson et al., 1990). Since this type of adjuvant treatment is generally well tolerated (Kaplan and Bagshaw, 1992; Lange et al., 1990; Stein et al., 1992), it seems, at least, justifiable.

Prostate cancer was clinically not only understaged, it was also considerably undergraded. Using the Dhom grading system, overall, 41 % of histological grades in the radical prostatectomy specimen were correctly predicted by either TURP, FNA or biopsy (Table 10). On the other hand, overgrading did not occur in a single case. In two smaller series, Haeggman et al. (1993) found that preoperative tumor grading by FNA, TURP or biopsy was in agreement with postoperative grading in the prostatectomy specimens in 48 % and 67 % of cases, respectively. When comparing the three different grading procedures, FNA had the highest false-negative rate (18 %). In a study of 335 specimens, the false-negative rate for FNA was 28 % (Stilmant et al., 1989). Ever since Franzen et al. (1960) introduced their technique of cytological diagnosis of prostatic tumors, controversy prevailed as to whether FNA was superior to biopsy with respect to more accuracy and less morbidity (Chodak et al., 1984; Ekman et al., 1967; Knoenagel and Hauri, 1984). However, this controversy has been solved through the advent of TRUS-guided biopsies (Hodge et al., 1989a). A spring-loaded “Biopty“ device with a 18-gauge Tru-cut needle provides 15 mm cores for histological examination. This procedure is not more painful for the patient than FNA and complications (bleeding, infections) are minimal (Hammerer and Huland, 1994). TRUS guided biopsies are more sensitive than FNA in detecting cancer (Ragde et al., 1988) and provide valuable information about the spatial distribution of the cancer and a better representation of the true histological grade of the whole tumor (Stamey and

McNeal, 1992). At our institution, TRUS-guided biopsies were introduced in 1989 and have completely replaced FNA and finger-guided biopsies.

When we started this series of radical prostatectomies in 1976, we wanted to evaluate the outcome of the operation in clinically localized prostate cancer (N0) and, thus, did not

When we started this series of radical prostatectomies in 1976, we wanted to evaluate the outcome of the operation in clinically localized prostate cancer (N0) and, thus, did not preclude cases with positive lymph nodes on frozen sections (pN1-2) from radical prostatectomy. Therefore, there were as many as 35 % of patients with lymph node metastases on permanent sections. What are the preoperative criteria to define patients in whom staging lymph node dissection might not be necessary? As seen from Table 11, DRE is not very helpful to predict the side of nodal involvement. If lymphadenectomy had been performed only on the side with positive DRE, 7 of 38 cases (18 %) with pN1-2 status would have been missed. Nseyo and Pontes (1989) studied intraprostatic tumor location and pelvic lymph node metastatic pattern in a small series of 12 patients. Seven of the 12 patients (58 %) with stage D1 disease had bilateral pelvic lymph node metastases as compared to 13 of 38 patients (34 %) in our series (Table 11). They found that all patients with unilateral intraprostatic tumor had either ipsilateral or bilateral lymph node metastases and that there were no cases in which contralateral nodal involvement occured without tumor also involving the pelvic lymph nodes ipsilateral to the intraprostatic tumor site. Clinically of more importance, Daniels and colleagues (1992) analyzed patients with tumors digitally localized to 1 prostatic lobe who underwent random systematic TRUS biopsies of both lobes. The likelihood for nodal disease was 8 % in patients with bilaterally positive biopsies compared to 0 % in patients with unilaterally positive biopsies. Hammerer et al. (1992) performed TRUS guided mapping of the prostate with six random systematic biopsies in patients who subsequently underwent pelvic lymphadenectomy. If only 1 or 2 of the 6 core biopsies were positive for prostate cancer, no lymph node metastases could be found; whereas if 5 or 6 of the 6 cores were involved, two thirds of the patients had lymph node metastases.

Using PSA as a parameter for predicting lymph node metastases, we found that only 1 of 11 patients (9 %) with a PSA value below the cut-off level of 12 ng/ml had positive findings (Table 13). The lowest PSA in a patient with nodal involvement was 8 ng/ml. Stamey et al. (1989), by using the same polyclonal assay, found that no patient with a PSA below 10 ng/ml had lymph node metastases. For the monoclonal Hybritech assay also, Sassine and Schulman (1993) could not detect positive lymph nodes in patients with a PSA of less than 10 ng/ml and in the series of Oesterling et al. (1988), none of the patients with nodal involvement had a preoperative PSA concentration in the normal range.

To conclude from our series and from the literature, clinical understaging and – to a lesser extent – undergrading are the major problems in the selection of patients for radical prostatectomy. DRE is completely insufficient for prediction of organ-confined cancer. PSA values over 30 ng/ml (Yang assay) and over 20 ng/ml (Hybritech assay), respectively are highly suspicious for extraprostatic disease. PAP does not add any valuable information and should be abandoned. Staging lymphadenectomy can probably be omitted in patients with a PSA in the normal range and in patients with TRUS guided random systematic biopsies depending on the number of positive cores.

IV. Prognostic factors based on long-term follow-up

4.1 Tumor volume*

As delineated in chapter 2.3., quantitated tumor volume is the single most important prognostic factor in the individual patient with carcinoma of the prostate. Indeed, members of the American Cancer Society and the European Organization for Research and Treatment of Cancer (EORTC) have proposed to use tumor volume as an adjunct to the official TNM staging system (Bostwick et al., 1993). However, exact determination of tumor volume preoperatively is not yet possible and serial step-sectioning of radical prostatectomy specimens for measuring tumor volume postoperatively is expensive and not suitable for daily pathological routine. There is a practical need for an abbreviated standard procedure for accurate tumor volume estimation in the radical prostatectomy specimen.

Currently, with more than 700 patients in the Stanford series, it has been possible to use cancer volume to define at least three risk levels for nodal metastasis, poorly differentiated tumor, seminal vesicle invasion, and capsule penetration. All variables correlate strongly with three cancer volume categories. Patients with less than 4 cc of cancer were almost invariably favorable for all morphologic variables and were thought to be cured; increasing volumes between 4 cc and 12 cc were associated with worsening prognostic indicators; all patients with more than 12 cc of cancer have had either positive margins or metastases. It should be noted that these findings are limited to clinical stage A and B patients with at most microscopic nodal metastasis; patients with known distant metastases or larger nodal metastases were excluded from radical prostatectomy.

Similar techniques for quantitative evaluation of prostate cancer volume are now in use at other centers (Partin et al., 1989; Wheeler, 1989); however, time, expense, and labor make the serial blocking and mapping of prostate specimens impractical for general use. A more simplified procedure is needed, and several have been proposed (Hall et al., 1991; Humphrey and Vollmer, 1990), but they were designed primarily for convenience and not tested for reliability and accuracy of volume estimation by comparison with alternate procedures and by ranking against a more quantitative standard.

Accordingly, we tested the accuracy of several abbreviated sectioning and mapping modifications of the Stanford technique; these modifications require fewer than half the standard number of slides. Slides were selected from previously mapped cases according to several abbreviated protocols, and the cancer was estimated on each by eye using a millimeter grid. Estimated volume by each protocol was then validated against the computer volume previously obtained from study of the complete set of slides.

To facilitate the efficient execution of the optimum abbreviated protocol, we designed a simple prostate slicing device to perform the sequence of cuts needed to obtain the appropriate slides. The device was tested on several prostates, and the time needed to perform the complete sectioning operation was determined.

* Poster Prize of the German Urological Association 1992

4.1.1 Materials and methods

Between January 1989 and August 1990, 145 radical prostatectomy specimens obtained at the Department of Urology at Stanford University were mapped and volumed as part of our clinical prostate cancer series. The series contained 109 stage B (rectally palpated) cancers (Figure 17). The other 36 tumors were not palpable but were detected either incidentally at transurethral resection (stage A, 13 cases), by transrectal ultrasound (TRUS, eight cases) or by an elevated serum prostate specific antigen (PSA, 15 cases).

The present study is based mainly on 102 stage B carcinomas in which the side of the tumor could be determined preoperatively by palpation. These tumors were substaged by the Stanford clinical classification (Stamey et al., 1988). There were 43 stage B 1 tumors in which the palpable nodule occupied less than half of one lobe. In 41 stage B 2 cancers, the nodule extended for more than half the distance from apex to base of one lobe, up to one entire lobe. B 3 tumors (six cases) represented either a lesion crossing the midline or separate nodules bilaterally, one being distinctively larger than the other. The remaining 12 tumors were not substaged explicitly and are referred here as B X.

All specimens initially had been processed and analyzed by the Stanford technique (see chapter 2.3.1. for detailed description). The present study deals with total cancer volume rather than manifest (largest) tumor volume and incidental tumor volumes (for prostates with more than one cancer), because with the elimination of slides it is no longer possible to distinguish between the largest cancer and possible incidental cancers.

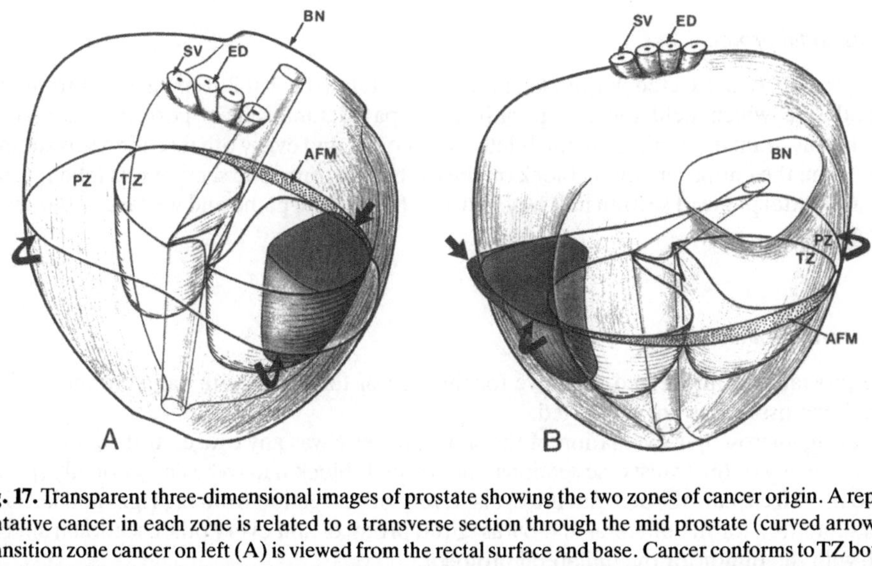

Fig. 17. Transparent three-dimensional images of prostate showing the two zones of cancer origin. A representative cancer in each zone is related to a transverse section through the mid prostate (curved arrows). Transition zone cancer on left (A) is viewed from the rectal surface and base. Cancer conforms to TZ boundary but invades anteriorly into anterior fibromuscular stroma (arrow). Non-transition zone cancer on right (B) is viewed from anterior surface. Cancer conforms to TZ boundary but invades posterolaterally through the capsule (arrow) in the region where nerve penetration of capsule is common. TZ, transition zone. PZ, peripheral zone. AFM, anterior fibromuscular stroma. B, bladder neck. ED, ejaculatory duct. SV, seminal vesicle (from: McNeal et al., 1990a).

The average weight of the 102 prostates was 51.8 grams (range 21.8 – 202.0). The mean height as measured from apex to base was 4.1 cm (range 2.5 – 7.4). The average width from left lateral to right lateral side was 4.8 cm (range 3.6 – 7.6). The mean thickness from rectal surface to the most anterior point (anterior fibromuscular stroma or benign hyperplastic nodules) was 3.8 cm (range 2.5 – 6.1). Without knowing the original computer calculated cancer volumes, original slides were reviewed and cancer volumes were estimated according to three sectioning and calculating protocols as presented below. For all three protocols, the anterior portion of the prostate (P-sections) was amputated at 3 cm from the rectal surface and parallel to it, as in the standard Stanford protocol. The apex of the prostate was also sectioned and subsectioned exactly as described in chapter 2.3.1. for the Stanford technique, with the exception that a 6 mm thick block was cut instead of a 5 mm block. The remaining main portion of the prostate was processed differently, as described below. The following descriptions represent measurements performed on the slides, but they are described as they would be executed in sectioning a fresh prostate.

Bilateral protocol

The prostate was bisected perpendicular to the rectal surface in a near-sagittal plane at 2.5 cm distance from one lateral side. If the prostate was more than 5 cm wide, a second cut was performed at 2.5 cm distance from the other lateral side. In this case, the remaining middle portion was not submitted for evaluation. Then, both lateral portions were serially blocked at 3 mm intervals in transverse planes parallel to the already amputated apical section and all the way up to the base. Only every other section on both sides was submitted for histological examination, starting with the second one above the apex.

Parasagittal protocol

The prostate was bisected perpendicular to the rectal surface at 2.5 cm distance from that lateral side which held the preoperatively palpated tumor. This portion was serially blocked at 3 mm intervals, as in the bilateral protocol, and every other section was submitted. From the entire remaining block on the other side, only one section was taken, using a parasagittal plane of section half way between the sagittal plane and the lateral border of the gland.

Unilateral protocol

The prostate was processed as above for the side of the gland with palpable tumor. The remaining tissue was not submitted.

During microscopic evaluation of the slides, if there was any cancer at the anterior cut border of any of the transverse sections, the whole P-block had to be cut coronally (parallel to the 3.0 cm cut-off) at 3 mm intervals. Every other section from the right and left side was submitted for the bilateral and parasagittal protocol and every other section from the side with the tumor for the unilateral protocol.

Total cancer volume was calculated as follows: on each slide all areas with cancer were outlined precisely with ink dots under the microscope using low magnification. Each slide containing tumor was placed on a grid of ruled lines on white paper. Tumor area was estimated from the number of grid squares within the ink-dotted cancer boundary. For convenience of estimation, grid lines were spaced 4 mm apart both vertically and horizontally (4 mm squares = 16 square mm).

Then each cancer area was multiplied by its appropriate thickness factor and by a factor of 1.5 for tissue shrinkage during processing (Figure 18). For the transverse sections, this

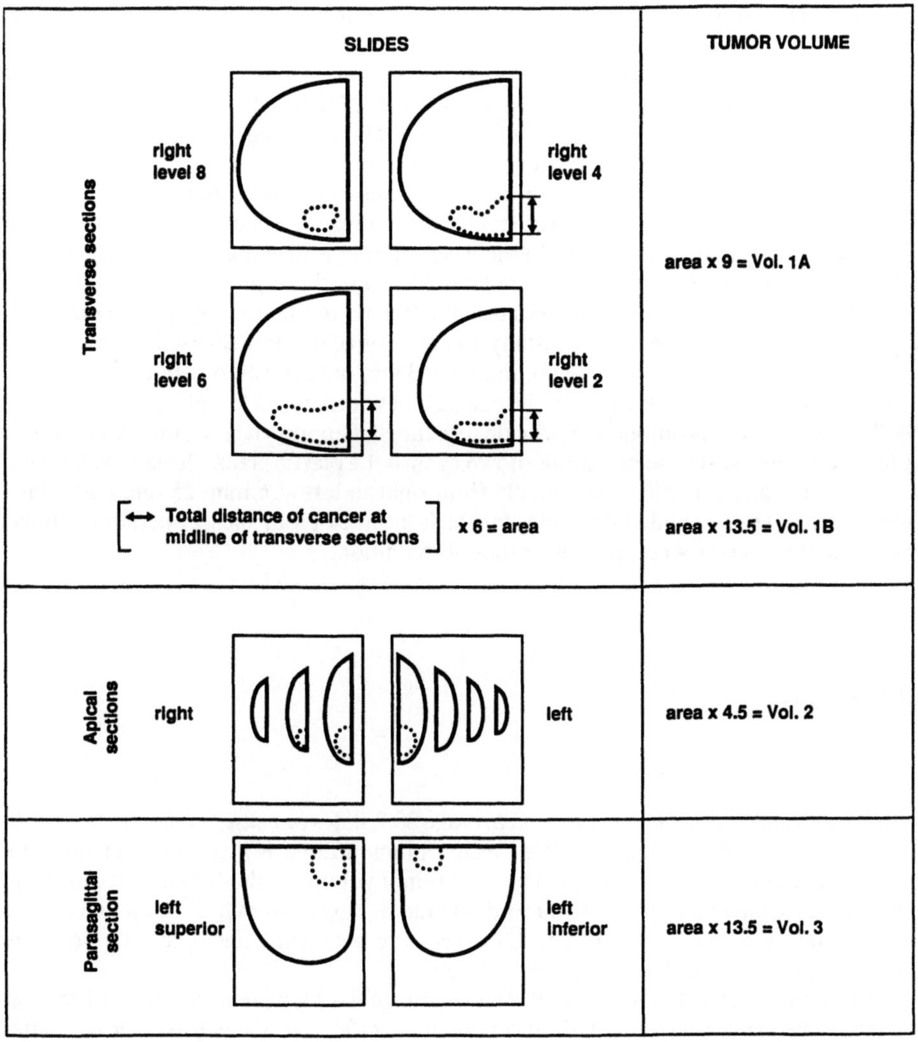

Fig. 18. Parasagittal abbreviated sectioning protocol. Typical case with a total of eight slides. Boundaries of the prostate are marked with a solid line. Areas of cancer are outlined with ink dots. Four transverse sections are displayed (levels 2, 4, 6, 8) from the right side with the preoperatively palpated tumor. The entire apex was cut sagittally at 3 mm intervals and divided into right and left. From the contralateral (left) side of the prostate, one parasagittal section was obtained and divided into two (superior and inferior) to accommodate the dimensions of microscopic slides. See text for tumor volume calculation (from: Schmid and McNeal, 1992).

factor was 9 (6 x 1.5), for the apical sections it was 4.5 (3 x 1.5) and for the parasagittal section it was 13.5 (9 x 1.5).

For the parasagittal protocol, additional information could be gained from each transverse slide, depending on the amount of cancer that had been transsected at the midline. This area was calculated by summing the lengths of the cut tumor edge at the prostate bisection margin on each transverse section and multiplying the sum by 6 to obtain an area. This calculated area then was multiplied by 13.5 (9 x 1.5). Adding all subvolumes yielded the total cancer volume. There were two subvolumes (transverse and apical sections) for the bilateral and unilateral protocols and four subvolumes for the parasagittal protocol (Figure 18).

For all three protocols, if there were P-sections, all tumor areas on these P-sections were multiplied by a factor of 9 (6 x 1.5). Stage A cases, TRUS-detected cancers and PSA-detected cancers were finally reviewed in light of findings for stage B tumors, and suggestions were made for abbreviated protocols in these cases also.

A slicing device was designed to use with the optimum protocol, but adaptable for all. The three abbreviated sectioning protocols and the original Stanford protocol had four basic slicing operations in common. In the order of most efficient execution they were as follows: a) amputation of anterior tissue (P-sections) in those prostates which were too thick for a single transverse section because of BPH; b) amputation of apical block of tissue, to be later subsectioned parasagittally; c) bisection of prostate sagittally into right and left halves; and d) serial transverse sectioning at 3 mm of each half prostate.

A knife guide was built of clear acrylic plastic blocks cemented to a plastic plate (Figure 19). The blocks were positioned to provide a channel of appropriate width to accomodate a prostate resting with its rectal surface down against the plastic plate. Three gaps were left in the channel and arranged sequentially from right to left at 6 mm, 25 mm and 3 mm. These acted as spacers and knife guides for the last three of four slicing operations above. The sequence acted as a reminder for order of execution.

4.1.2 Results

Comparison of abbreviated protocols

With the original Stanford technique, on average 26.2 slides per case (range 16–67) had to be examined in order to calculate the cancer volume (Table 14); this number does not include sections for seminal vesicles. The total tumor volume of the 102 stage B cancers as determined by the computerized Stanford technique ranged from 0.25 cc up to 34.82 cc. Twenty-nine cases had less than 2 cc, 23 cases were between 2 and 4 cc, 31 cases were between 4 and 8 cc and 19 cases exceeded 8 cc.

With the bilateral technique, only 11.7 slides (range 8 – 20) were necessary. In 102 stage B cancers, mean average estimated cancer volume was 94.2 % of mean average computer volume obtained with the full set of slides. Of more importance, however, is the range of our estimates (Figure 20). Ninety-six percent of the cases were within ± 20 % of the computer volume.

With the parasagittal technique, 8.8 slides (range 6 – 15) were necessary. Mean average estimated cancer volume was 95.3 % of mean average computer volume obtained with the full set of slides. Of the cases, 89 % were within ± 20 % of the computer volume (Figure 21).

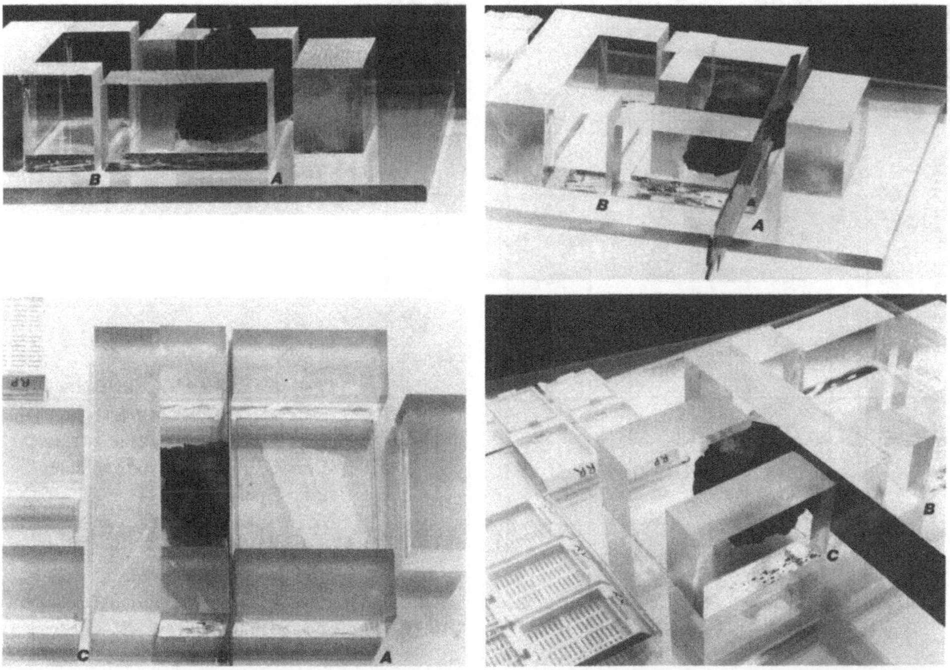

Fig. 19. Prostate slicing device. **(a)** Horizontal amputation of the anterior portion (P-sections). **(b)** Amputation of the apex at station A. **(c)** Bisection of the prostate at station B. The side with the tumor is pressed against the mid-transverse plastic block. **(d)** Slicing of the tissue block containing the tumor in transverse planes at station C. See text for details (from: Schmid and McNeal, 1992).

With the unilateral technique, 5.9 slides (range 4 – 10) were obtained; however, the unilateral technique proved to be clearly less accurate. Mean average estimated cancer volume was 74.8 % of mean average computer volume obtained with the full set of slides. Only 49 % of all estimates were within ± 20 % of the computer volume (Figure 22).

Table 14. Comparison of the three protocols with the Stanford technique[a]

	Stanford technique (computer)	Bilateral technique	Parasagittal technique	Unilateral technique
Slides per case				
Mean (%)	26.2 (100)	11.7 (45)	8.8 (34)	5.9 (23)
Range	16–67	8–20	6–15	4–10
Probability[b]	1.00	0.96	0.89	0.49

[a] Comparison was with regard to slides used for determination of total cancer volume and probability of being within a certain range of the computer-determined volume

[b] To be within 20 % of computer volume

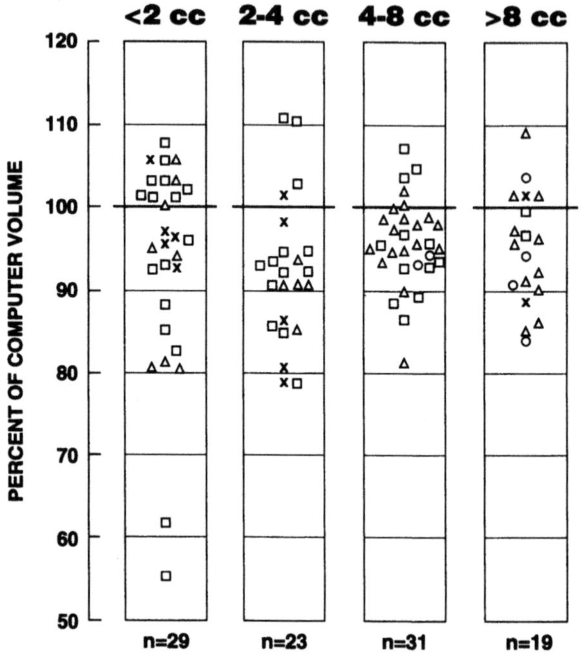

Fig. 20. Volume estimates by the bilateral technique expressed as percent of computer volume, which is stratified into four volume categories: □ stage B1 (n = 43), △ stage B2 (n = 41), ○ stage B3 (n = 6), × not determined (n = 12). The probability to be within ± 20 % of computer volume was 0.96 (from: Schmid and McNeal, 1992).

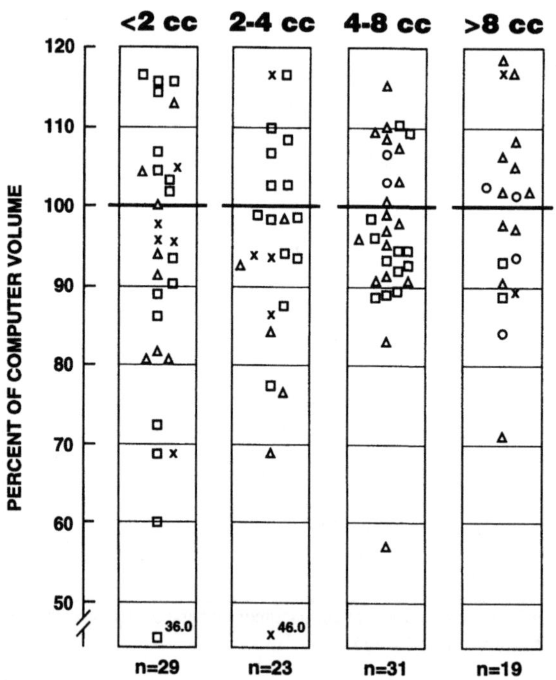

Fig. 21. Volume estimates by the parasagittal technique expressed as percent of computer volume, which is stratified into four volume categories. Cases are represented by the same symbols as in Figure 20. The probability to be within ± 20 % of computer volume was 0.89 (from: Schmid and McNeal, 1992).

Problems and modifications

Of 102 stage B cancers, in 63 cases there were anterior (P) sections because the thickness of the prostate exceeded 3.0 cm; but only 21 cases had tumor present in these P-sections. Therefore, in these 21 cases, we had to examine an additional average of 3 slides per case (range 1 – 6) for the bilateral and the parasagittal technique and 1.8 slides (range 1 – 3) for the unilateral technique. We did not find a single case with an isolated tumor in the P-sections that was not also identified at the anterior margin of the transverse sections. This was also true for the 36 nonpalpable cancers, except for one case with an incidental cancer of 0.03 cc, which was represented only in one P-section.

By inspection of the original tumor maps of the 36 nonpalpable cancers, the bilateral protocol yielded results similar to those for stage B cancers. The parasagittal protocol was not applicable, however, because the side of the tumor cannot be determined preoperatively in nonpalpable cancers.

For prostates more than 6 cm wide (four of 145 cases in this series), we suggest cutting off the P-section at 3 cm parallel to the rectal surface, and the apex at 6 mm perpendicular to the rectal surface free-handed; then proceed with the bilateral protocol.

The parasagittal technique assigned only four cases to a different volume risk category than the full Stanford technique using the 4 cc and 12 cc cutoff points. A 4.0 cc cancer was estimated at 3.6 cc, and a 4.8 cc cancer was estimated at 3.9 cc. Another carcinoma calculated at 11.9 cc by computer was estimated as 13.9 cc, and a 12.6 cc tumor was estimated as

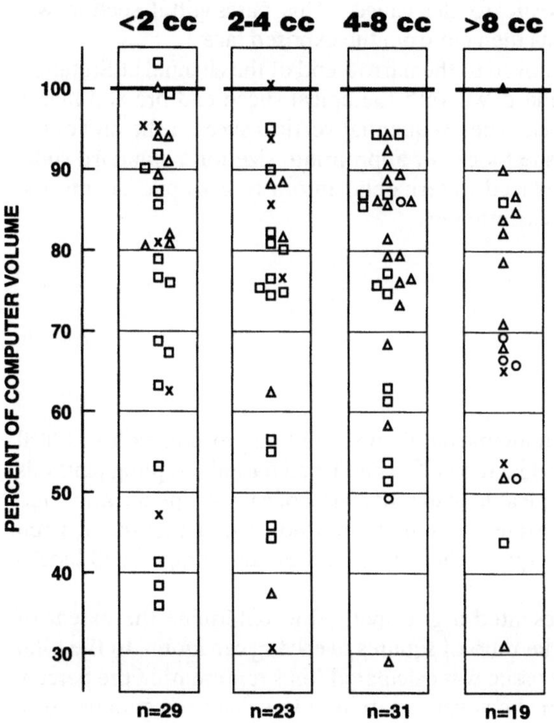

Fig. 22. Volume estimates by the unilateral technique expressed as percent of computer volume, which is stratified into four volume categories. Cases are represented by the same symbols as in Figure 20. The probability to be within ± 20 % of computer volume was 0.49 (from: Schmid and McNeal, 1992).

11.7 cc. Considering the arbitrary nature of these cutoff points, it is clear that in these four cases both the calculated and estimated values are close enough to the cutoff to be considered borderline.

Use of the device

Use of the slicing device in executing the parasagittal protocol was tested on 10 recent prostatectomy specimens. Average time for the complete procedure was 10 minutes. After amputation of the seminal vesicles, the prostate was placed with rectal surface down into the channel at its right end (Station A, Figure 19a). The prostate was oriented with its apical margin against the right transverse end block, so that the right side of the prostate rested against the near wall of the channel. The prostate was pressed lightly against the right end block with a movable plastic block. Then a horizontal slice along the top of the channel (Figure 19a) and a vertical slice at the end of the 6 mm gap (Figure 19b) amputated the anterior (P-sections) and apical tissues.

At Station B (Figure 19c), the apical sliced end of the prostate was held against the near wall of the channel for a right-sided cancer, or it was held against the far wall with the base on the near side for a left-sided cancer. With the prostate pressed lightly against the mid-transverse plastic block, a vertical slice would include the cancer side (left or right) in a 25 mm thick tissue block. This would be a sagittal cut of a 50 mm wide prostate. It would be a little more or less for a smaller or larger prostate, but it would always fit on a standard slide.

The 25 mm tissue block was removed and the contralateral prostate slid over across the gap, preserving the same orientation, until another slice through the same gap would bisect the side of the prostate opposite to the cancer. This parasagittal section was estimated by eye and a 3 mm block was then cut from the exposed face.

The 25 mm block with cancer was moved to the narrow end of the channel at Station C (Figure 19d) and positioned rectal side down with the apical sliced end pressed lightly against the mid-transverse plastic block. Then sequential vertical slices at the end of the 3 mm gap created 3 mm finished tissue blocks of appropriate size for a standard slide. Each tissue block, when sliced was placed (alternately) into a reserve pile or into the appropriately labelled cassette in the cassette rack.

4.1.3 Discussion

Only very few reports exist on systematic partial tissue sampling procedures for radical prostatectomy specimens. Hall and colleagues (1991) described partial sampling methods that focus on gross cancer, and they were able to identify 96 % of capsular penetration and 84 % of positive margins in stage B prostates examined with whole mount sections at 6 mm (roughly similar to our bilateral technique). Their method used an average of 13 blocks (range 7 – 36) per case.

Humphrey and Vollmer (1990) presented a grid method to determine the extent of tumor in prostatectomy specimens. The ratio of squares overlying carcinoma to the total number of squares overlying prostate tissue was calculated, thus representing the percentage of the prostate involved by tumor; however, no attempt was made to estimate absolute tumor volume. Furthermore, the substantial spread of grid ratio values made it difficult to predict, in an individual case, clinical local recurrence or the appearance of metastatic tumor.

Our previous experience in correlating volume with other morphologic and clinical variables lead us to believe that an error of volume estimate of ± 20 % is acceptable. The optimum predictive information is gained by classifying tumors as less than 4 cc, 4 to 12 cc or more than 12 cc. Thus, both the bilateral and parasagittal techniques yield excellent results (Table 14). The unilateral technique, however, is distinctively worse and cannot be recommended.

We did not quantitate the effect of abbreviated sectioning on estimation of positive margins or capsule penetration; however, the area of greatest susceptibility to positive margins was left intact in the abbreviated protocols. Capsule penetration has been shown to have relatively little influence on prognosis independent of cancer volume and grade. Also, only areas of capsule penetration greater than 0.5 square cm appear related to prognosis at all (McNeal et al., 1990a). Hence, although we did not quantitate the effect of the abbreviated protocols on determination of margins or capsule penetration, we feel that reduction in accuracy in this area is relatively slight, and the procedure is superior to those in which sections are taken without a standard protocol.

The accuracy of our estimates, regardless of the technique used (bilateral, parasagittal, unilateral), did not depend on the absolute amount of tumor volume. For each of the four categories (< 2 cc, 2 – 4 cc, 4 – 8 cc, and > 8 cc), we found similar results, although there was a slight tendency for more accurate estimates toward higher volumes (Figures 20, 21, 22).

About 70 % of all radical prostatectomy specimens can be processed by the parasagittal technique, including all stage B cancers in which the side of the nodule can be determined clearly as well as some prostates with clearly defined ultrasound lesions. For the other 30 % of cases in which the side of the tumor is unknown (i.e., stage A, PSA-detected cancers, some TRUS-detected cancers and cases with bilateral firmness and "bilateral" stage B 3, respectively), we recommend the bilateral abbreviated technique.

In summary, our findings define a simple and relatively inexpensive procedure for deriving important prognostic information in a systematic fashion from the morphologic data obtained in prostatectomy specimens for adenocarcinoma of the prostate.

4.2 Conventional morphology

From the Basel series of 140 patients (see chapter 3.1.), eight were not evaluable for long-term follow-up. Seven patients were excluded because they received immediate orchiectomy due to grossly involved pelvic lymph nodes (pN2) and one patient was excluded because of chemotherapy for lung cancer. For the remaining 132 patients, mean follow-up was 97 months (8 years 1 month), median follow-up was 86 months (7 years 2 months), with a range of 12 – 212 months (1 year – 17 years 8 months).

Follow-up examinations at our clinic were performed every three months during the first year, every six months during the second year and yearly thereafter. They consisted of physical examination with digital rectal examination (DRE), determination of PSA, PAP, alkaline phosphatase, creatinine and erythrocyte sedimentation rate and chest X-ray. Biopsy of the anastomosis and bone scans were performed if any of the above examinations were suspicious for relapse. Progression of disease was defined as follows: appearance of biopsy proven local recurrence, appearance of distant metastases on chest X-rays or bone scans, elevation of PSA, PAP or alkaline phosphatase above the normal range and increasing values of PSA or PAP within the normal ranges of up to 12 ng/ml and up to 3.1 ng/ml, respectively.

Statistical analysis was based on the actuarial method of Kaplan and Meier (1958). Curves representing nonparametric estimates of interval to first evidence of treatment failure (disease free survival, DFS) and interval to cause-specific death (corrected overall survival, COS) were generated. The association of nominal factors with survival, i.e. the comparison between different subgroups of prognostic factors, was done using the log-rank test (Mantel, 1966).

Radical prostatectomy specimens were processed as follows: the specimen was weighed and measured and then immersed in 4 % formalin overnight. The entire prostate was serially blocked at 3 μm intervals from apex to base in transverse sections perpendicular to the rectal surface and the distal urethra. Whole mount sections were processed into paraffin, and slides were cut at 5 μm and stained with hematoxylin/eosin and v. Gieson-stain.

4.2.1 Histological grade

The Dhom grading system (Dhom, 1977; Mueller et al., 1980) was applied to the radical prostatectomy specimens. The worst grade in all whole mount sections was determined by a single pathologist.

Ten years after surgery, 61 % of patients with grade 1, 44 % of patients with grade 2, and 40 % of patients with grade 3 were free of disease (Figure 23). The differences between dis-

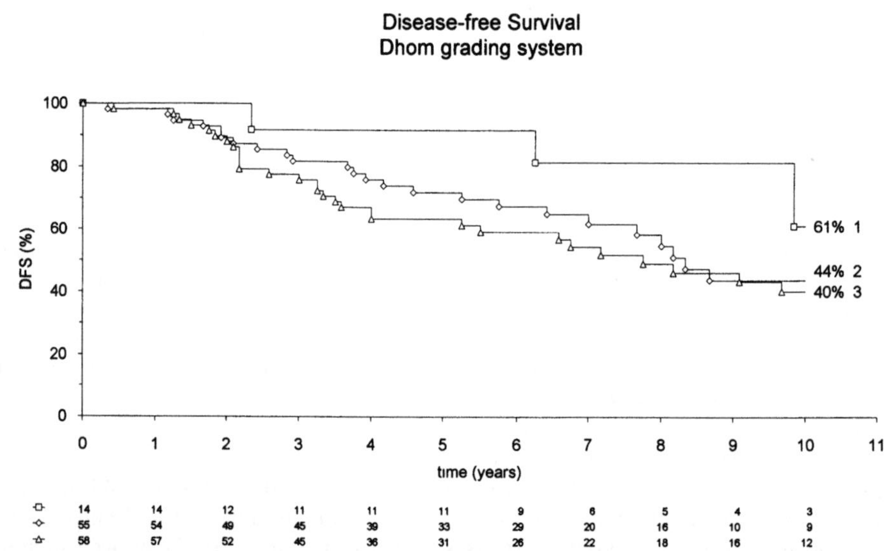

Fig. 23. Probability of not failing as function of histological grade (Dhom grades 1 – 3).

ease-free survival curves did not reach statistical significance (p = 0.171 for grade 1 versus grade 2; p = 0.092 for grade 1 versus grade 3; and p = 0.484 for grade 2 versus grade 3). The probability of not dying from prostate cancer after ten years was 89 % for grade 1, 77 % for grade 2, and 65 % for grade 3 (Figure 24). Again, the differences between survival curves were statistically not significant (p = 0.535 for grade 1 versus grade 2; p = 0.155 for grade 1 versus grade 3; and p = 0.087 for grade 2 versus grade 3).

These findings were somewhat surprising since histological grade is a well established prognostic factor in prostate cancer (Helpap, 1989; Stamey and McNeal, 1992). A possible explanation could be that most patients belonged to pT2 and early pT3 category. They were in a relatively small tumor volume range, where grade might be less helpful when compared to the entire spectrum of prostate cancer. In prostate cancer there is almost always a heterogeneity of grades in the same tumor, with progressing dedifferentiation in higher tumor volumes (Cumming et al., 1990; McNeal et al., 1986; Schmassmann and Mihatsch, 1983). In fact, McNeal and colleagues (1990) could convincingly show that the absolute amount of undifferentiated grades gave the most information on prognosis in the individual patient. As a conclusion, we recommend to quantify each histological grade in radical prostatectomy specimens.

Finally, it is interesting to compare our results to a recent large series of untreated patients. Chodak et al. (1994) pooled and analyzed six nonrandomized studies on patients with clinically localized prostate cancer who were managed conservatively. The disease-specific survival after ten years was 87 % for patients with histological grade 1 and 2; this number is similar to that of our radical prostatectomy treated patients with grade 1 and 2 (Figure 24). However, disease-specific survival rates dropped to 34 % in untreated patients with grade 3; while in our series 65 % of patients with grade 3 were still alive. It is clear that these comparisons should be interpreted with caution, but they might suggest that some patients with clinically localized prostate cancer and grade 1 or 2 could be managed conservatively while patients with grade 3 do better with a radical prostatectomy.

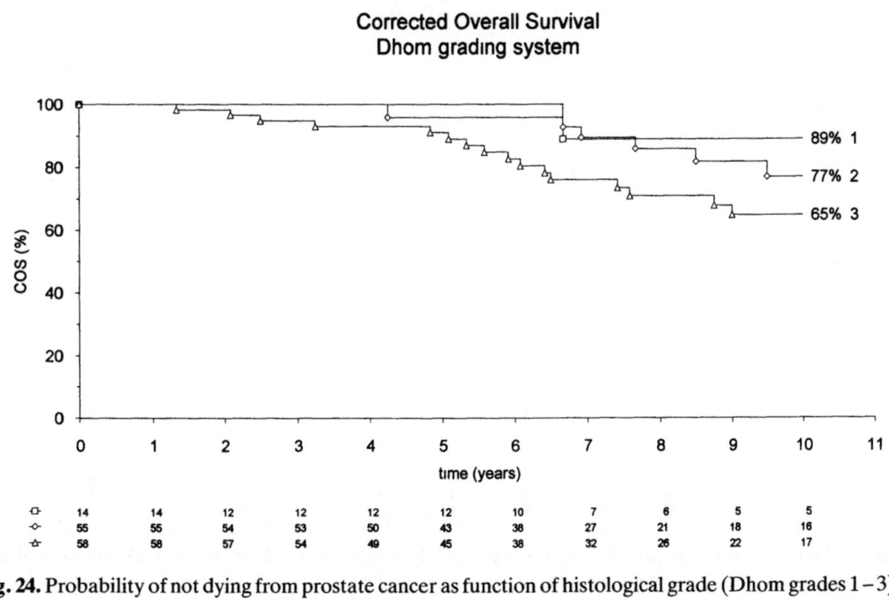

Fig. 24. Probability of not dying from prostate cancer as function of histological grade (Dhom grades 1–3).

4.2.2 Capsular involvement

To study the impact of microinvasion of the prostatic capsule, pathological category pT3 was further divided into pT3.1 (invasion of the capsule) and pT3.2 (penetration of the capsule with tumor extension beyond). For this purpose, all histological slides were re-examined by a single pathologist.

Ten years after radical prostatectomy, 100 % of patients in category pT1-2, 66 % of patients in category pT3.1, and 31 % of patients in category pT3.2 were free from relapse (Figure 25). The differences between disease-free survival curves were statistically significant ($p = 0.042$ for pT1-2 versus pT3.1; $p = 0.000$ for pT1-2 versus pT3.2; and $p = 0.007$ for pT3.1 versus pT3.2). The cause-specific survival at ten years was 100 % for pT1-2, 90 % for pT3.1, and 63 % for pT3.2 (Figure 26). The curves between category pT1-2 and pT3.1 did not differ significantly ($p = 0.311$). However, there were significant differences between pT1-2 and pT3.2 ($p = 0.040$) and between pT3.1 and pT3.2 ($p = 0.037$).

In a previous study from our institution, Hering et al. (1990) could demonstrate that only complete penetration of the prostatic capsule did adversely affect prognosis of radical prostatectomy treated patients. The present series with an extended follow-up again could confirm these data. There was a significant difference between patients in category pT3.1 versus pT3.2 with regard to DFS (Figure 25) and COS (Figure 26), respectively. Reports from other groups are in keeping with these findings (Eggleston and Walsh, 1985; McNeal et al., 1986; Mukamel et al., 1990; Stamey et al., 1988; Van den Ouden et al., 1992).

Previous studies of perineural space invasion by cancer presumed that it represented perineural lymphatic invasion but more recent work has shown that there are no lymphatics within the perineurium (Rodin et al., 1967) and that most penetration of the capsule by prostate cancer is facilitated spread represented by extension of cancer through the capsule along conduits provided by the perineural spaces (Mihatsch, 1994; Villers et al.,

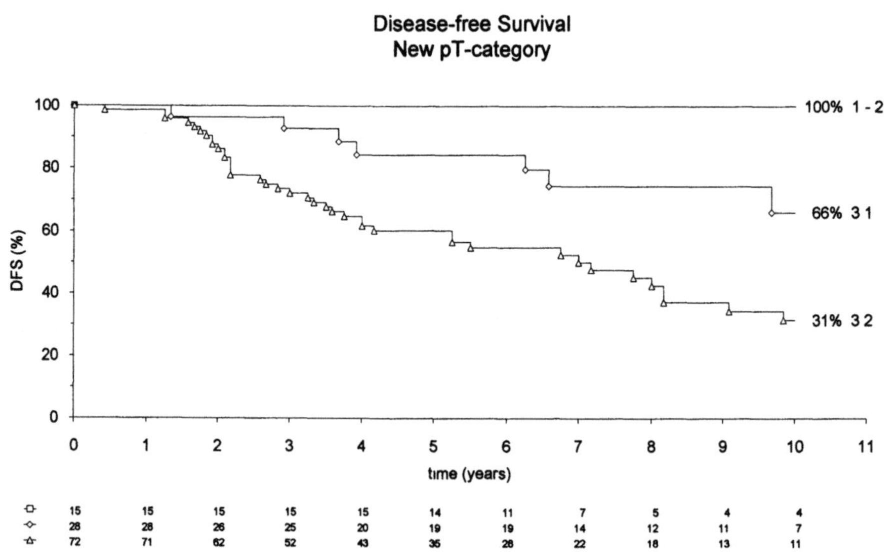

Fig. 25. Freedom from relapse according to completely organ-confined cancer (pT1-2), invasion of the prostatic capsule (pT3.1) and penetration of the capsule (pT3.2).

1989). An exception is the medial posterior area of the prostate, where tumor can progress within Denonvillier's fascia unrelated to perineural space invasion (Villers et al., 1993). In general, the area of highest susceptibility for capsular penetration and positive margins is the apex of the prostate (Stamey et al., 1989; Voges et al., 1992).

When comparing categories pT1-2 to pT3.1, we found a discrepancy between DFS (Figure 25; p = 0.042) and COS (Figure 26; p = 0.311). A conclusion would be to cut additional slides in specimens with invasion of the capsule. This would allow to truly exclude capsule penetration and assign patients to category pT1-2, or to discover capsule penetration in these additional slides and assign patients to category pT3.2.

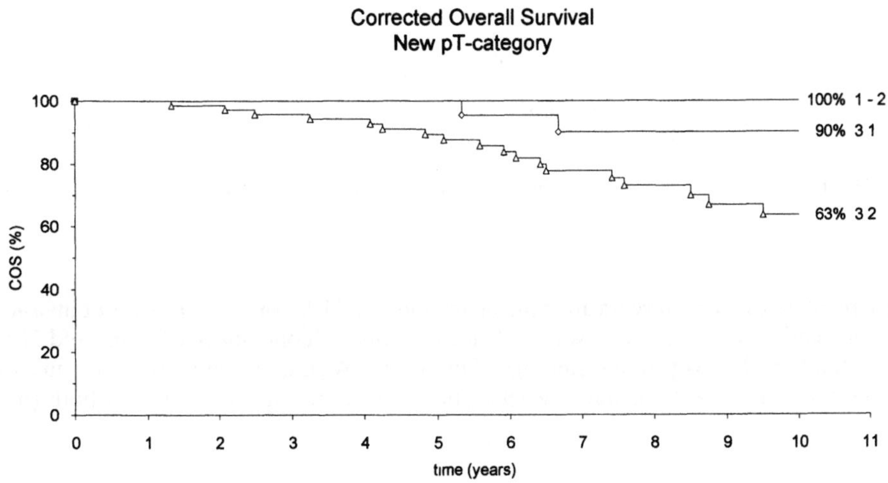

	0	1	2	3	4	5	6	7	8	9	10
□	15	15	15	15	15	14	11	7	5	4	4
◇	28	28	27	27	24	23	21	17	14	13	10
△	72	72	69	66	61	52	43	34	27	21	18

Fig. 26. Cause-specific survival according to completely organ-confined cancer (pT1-2), invasion of the prostatic capsule (pT3.1) and penetration of the capsule (pT3.2).

4.2.3 Seminal vesicle invasion

The seminal vesicles were cut in a coronal plane, i.e. longitudinally from base to apex, at 3 mm intervals. Statistical analysis was based on the number of tumor invaded seminal vesicles.

Ten years after the operation, 60 % of patients with negative seminal vesicles, 37 % of patients with invasion of one seminal vesicle, and 10 % of patients with invasion of both seminal vesicles were alive without evidence of treatment failure (Figure 27). The differences between negative seminal vesicles and invasion of one (p = 0.006) or both (p = 0.000) seminal vesicles, respectively were statistically significant. There was no significance, however, when patients with one positive seminal vesicle were compared to patients with two positive seminal vesicles (p = 0.102). The probability of not having died

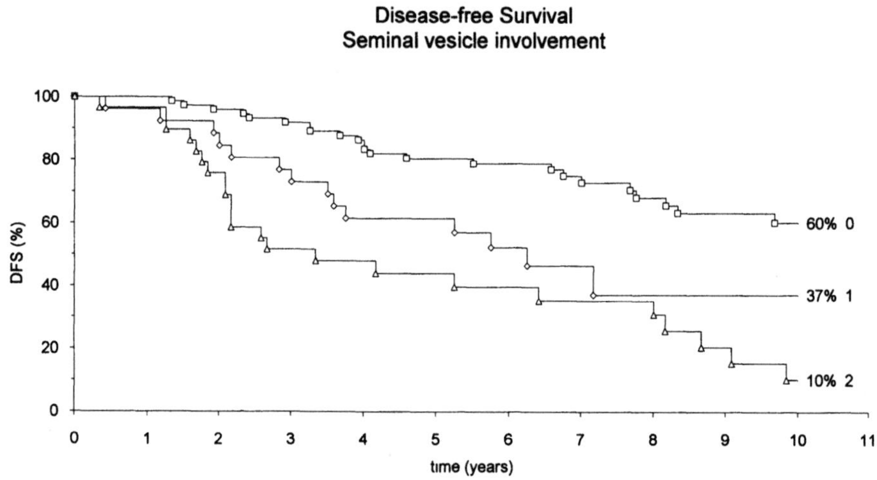

	0	1	2	3	4	5	6	7	8	9	10
□	76	76	71	68	61	51	46	36	28	23	19
◇	26	25	23	20	15	14	10	5	4	4	4
△	29	28	22	15	12	11	9	8	8	4	2

Fig. 27. Absence of treatment failure as function of number of invaded seminal vesicles.

from prostate cancer ten years after the operation was 83 % for patients without invasion of their seminal vesicles, and it was 56 % for patients with one positive finding and 51 % for patients with two positive findings (Figure 28). Again, the differences in survival curves between negative seminal vesicles and invasion of one (p = 0.013) or both (p =

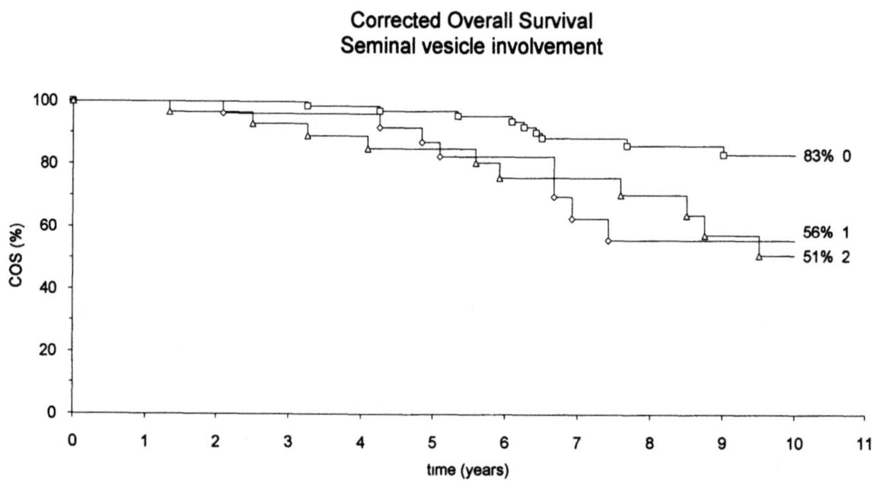

	0	1	2	3	4	5	6	7	8	9	10
□	76	76	73	73	69	62	56	44	35	31	26
◇	26	26	26	25	23	19	16	9	7	6	5
△	29	29	28	25	22	21	16	14	12	9	8

Fig. 28. Absence of death from prostate cancer as function of number of invaded seminal vesicles.

0.004) seminal vesicles, respectively were statistically significant. In contrast, patients with one positive seminal vesicle did not differ from patients with two positive seminal vesicles ($p = 0.951$).

Invasion of seminal vesicles has long been recognized as an index of poor prognosis (Jewett et al., 1972). However, since it represents a dichotomous variable, its true biological significance has not been fully appreciated. Indeed, our data shows that there is a considerable difference between patients with negative versus positive seminal vesicles with respect to DFS (Figure 27) and COS (Figure 28). Mukamel et al. (1990) obtained similar results in their comparable series. On the other hand, it did not matter if only one or both seminal vesicles were invaded.

Villers et al. (1990) and Wheeler (1989) stressed the importance of serially sectioning seminal vesicles and discussed different patterns of cancer spread from the prostate to the seminal vesicles. When quantifying seminal vesicle involvement, Villers et al. (1990) found that it represented a morphological reflection of biological tumor progression. However, other continuous variables like tumor volume and quantitative histological grade were stronger predictors of cancer dissemination as measured by the presence of lymph node metastases.

4.2.4 Extent of lymph node metastasis

To study the influence of minimal lymph node metastasis, category pN1 (metastasis in 1 unilateral lymph node) was divided into pN1.1 (micrometastasis in 1 unilateral lymph node with a diameter of 5 mm or less) and pN1.2 (unilateral in 1 lymph node with a diameter of more than 5 mm eventually visible macroscopically or palpable).

Ten years after surgery, 58 % of patients with negative lymph nodes, 37 % of patients in category pN1.1, 25 % of patients in category pN1.2, and 10 % of patients in category pN2 were free from relapse (Figure 29). The differences between time to progression Kaplan Meier curves were as follows: $p = 0.073$ for pN0 versus pN1.1; $p = 0.156$ for pN0 versus pN1.2; $p = 0.000$ for pN0 versus pN2; $p = 0.725$ for pN1.1 versus pN1.2; $p = 0.001$ for pN1.1 versus pN2; and $p = 0.091$ for pN1.2 versus pN2. Adjusted overall survival at ten years was 83 % for patients with negative lymph nodes, 73 % for patients in category pN1.1, 33 % for patients in category pN1.2, and 29 % for patients in category pN2 (Figure 30). The differences between cause-specific survival curves were as follows: $p = 0.178$ for pN0 versus pN1.1; $p = 0.048$ for pN0 versus pN1.2; $p = 0.000$ for pN0 versus pN2; $p = 0.441$ for pN1.1 versus pN1.2; $p = 0.043$ for pN1.1 versus pN2; and $p = 0.484$ for pN1.2 versus pN2.

Pelvic lymph node metastasis is regarded as a sign of tumor dissemination and is generally considered a situation that precludes patients from radical prostatectomy (Gibbons et al., 1984). Even a single microscopic metastatic focus in only one node is a hallmark of prostate cancer that is not curable by any treatment modality (Gervasi et al., 1989; Gibbons et al., 1984; Scardino, 1989; Smith and Middleton, 1985). In contrast to these findings, Lange and Narayan (1983) reported favorable outcome of patients with microscopically detectable lymph node metastases who underwent radical prostatectomy and adjuvant radiotherapy.

In a previous study from Basel, Hering and coworkers (1990) could demonstrate that microscopic involvement (micrometastasis with a diameter of 5 mm or less) of 1 unilateral lymph node did not adversely affect prognosis. These patients with positive nodes

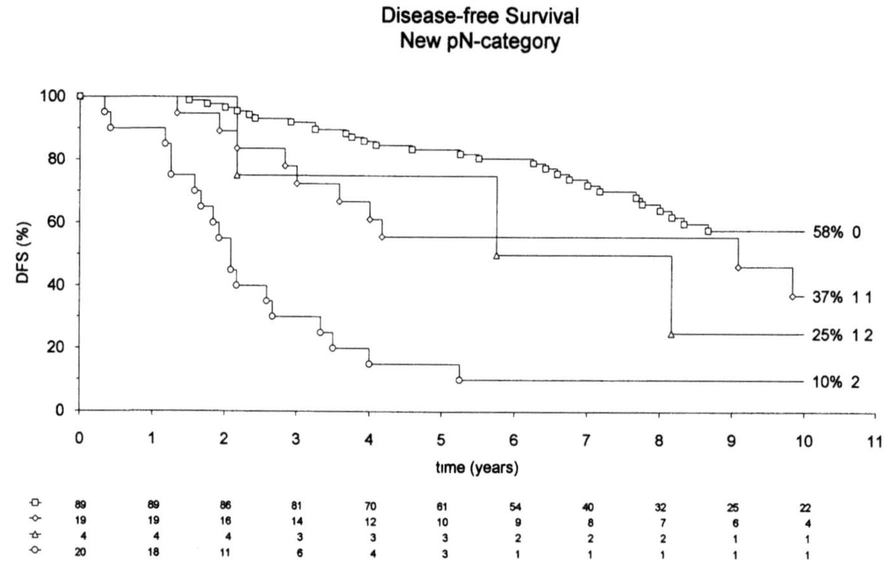

Fig. 29. Probability of not failing in relation to lymph node metastasis (see text for definition of pN1.1. and pN1.2).

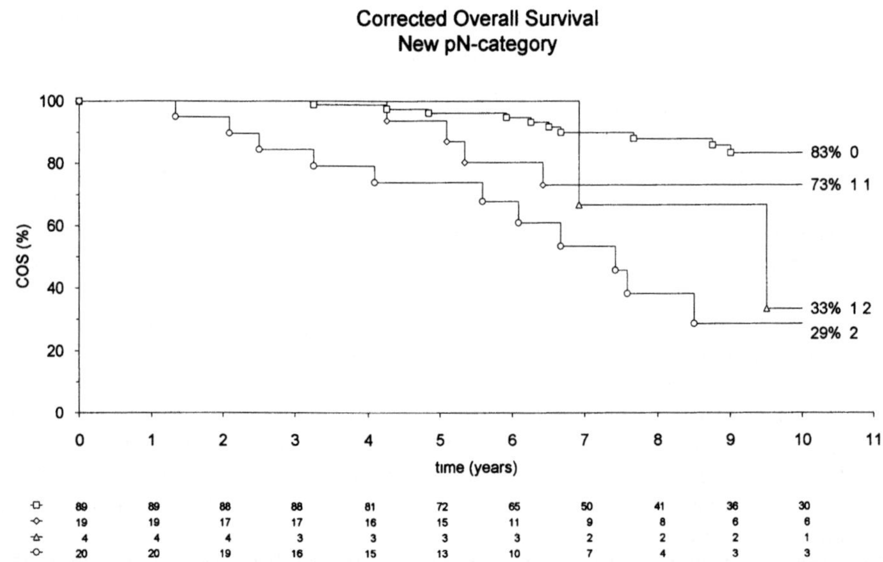

Fig. 30. Probability of not dying from prostate cancer in relation to lymph node metastasis (see text for definition of pN1.1 and pN1.2).

received adjuvant external beam irradiation. With more patients in the present series and a follow-up of additional four years, we again were able to confirm these findings. Disease-free survival curves (Figure 29) and corrected overall survival curves (Figure 30) did not differ for patients in category pN0 versus pN1.1. On the other hand, the differences for DFS and COS were statistically significant for patients in category pN1.1 versus pN2. As a preliminary conclusion, we suggest to perform radical prostatectomy and adjuvant radiotherapy in patients with minimal lymph node metastasis. However, in view of the prolonged natural history of prostate cancer, longer follow-up of these patients is needed.

4.3 Immunohistochemistry

A recent overview on histological and cytological characteristics of prostate cancer, on various cell kinetic methods and on cytogenetic as well as oncogenetic studies has been presented by Helpap (1993). In addition, there is growing evidence that cells from the APUD system (amine precursor uptake and decarboxylation) may play a role in prostate cancer. The APUD cells (neuroendocrine or endocrine-paracrine cells) of the prostate constitute, in addition to the basal and exocrine secretory cells, a third population of specialized epithelial cells. They probably subserve a paracrine or local regulatory role in prostatic growth and differentiation (Abrahamsson et al., 1986). Bonkhoff and colleagues (1991) found that proliferating prostatic acinar secretory cells in benign epithelium, demonstrated by Ki-67 immunoreactivity, were preferentially localized adjacent to neuroendocrine cells. These cells of the human prostate and urethra have been identified by various methods, predominantly silver stains and immunohistochemistry (di Sant'Agnese, 1988; di Sant'Agnese and de Mesy Jensen, 1987). They express, among other peptids, neuron-specific enolase (NSE) and Chromogranin A (CrGrA) which serve as marker substances.

NSE is an isoenzyme of the glycolytic enzyme enolase. It is present in the cytoplasm of all cells of the diffuse neuroendocrine system. CrGrA is a marker for endocrine cells that contain secretory granules (Lloyd and Wilson, 1983). It has been detected in pancreatic islet, adrenal medulla, thyroid C-cells, pituitary, parathyroid, enterochromaffin cells and tumors derived from these cells. NSE represents a highly sensitive marker of neuroendocrine cells, while CrGrA, although less sensitive, appears more specific (Abrahamsson et al., 1986).

The role of neuroendocrine cells as a prognostic factor in prostate cancer is under debate. There are but few studies in the literature and those were mainly performed on biopsy samples rather than on radical prostatectomy specimens, and long-term follow-up of patients is not reported. We therefore investigated the impact of the presence or absence of neuroendocrine cells in radical prostatectomy treated patients with respect to long-term prognosis.

4.3.1 Materials and methods

The material comprised 75 unselected radical prostatectomies from the Basel series. For immunohistochemistry selected tumor areas were dissected from the gross sections and re-embedded in paraplast. Five μm thick sections were treated according to standard techniques. Endogenous peroxidase activity was blocked with 3 % hydrogen peroxide in absolute methanol (30 min.). Non-specific binding was blocked by pre-incubation with normal serum of the species of the bridging antibody (dilution 1:10; 30 min.). The avidin-biotin-complex technique (Hsu et al., 1981) was employed using the ABC-elite kit (Vector, Burlingame, CA) according to the instructions of the supplier. The sections were incubated with the primary antibodies overnight at 4 degrees Celsius in a moist chamber. The immunoperoxidase was visualized with 3.3' diaminobenzidine (Serva, Chemie Brunnschwig, Basel/Switzerland). The intensity of the staining product was increased by treatment of the slides with 1 % osmium tetroxide for 2 min. The slides were counterstained with hematoxylin (Shandon), rehydrated and mounted in Eukitt (Kindler, Freiburg i.Br./Germany). Staining controls were carried out by replacing the primary antibody by PBS, verifying internal tissue controls and simultaneous staining of known positive tissue controls.

To demonstrate neuroendocrine cell types we used the mouse monoclonal antibody LK2H10 (Hybritech, San Diego, CA; 1:30000) against chromogranin-A (68000 daltons). In addition we used a mouse monoclonal antibody against human neuron-specific enolase (DAKO, Denmark; 1:6400) which reacts with human gamma-gamma enolase (46000 daltons).

The carcinomas were graded for neuroendocrine differentiation semiquantitatively as "negative" (0 %), "weak" (1 – 5 %; few scattered NE-positive tumor cells), and "moderate" (5 – 10 %; numerous NE-positive tumor cells).

The mean age of the 75 patients at time of surgery was 64.4 years, the median age was 65 years, and the range was 49 to 76 years. The patients were followed according to the criteria described in chapter 4.2. The mean follow-up was 90 months (7 years 6 months), the median follow-up was 80 months (6 years 8 months), and the range was 23 – 170 months (1 year 11 months – 14 years 2 months).

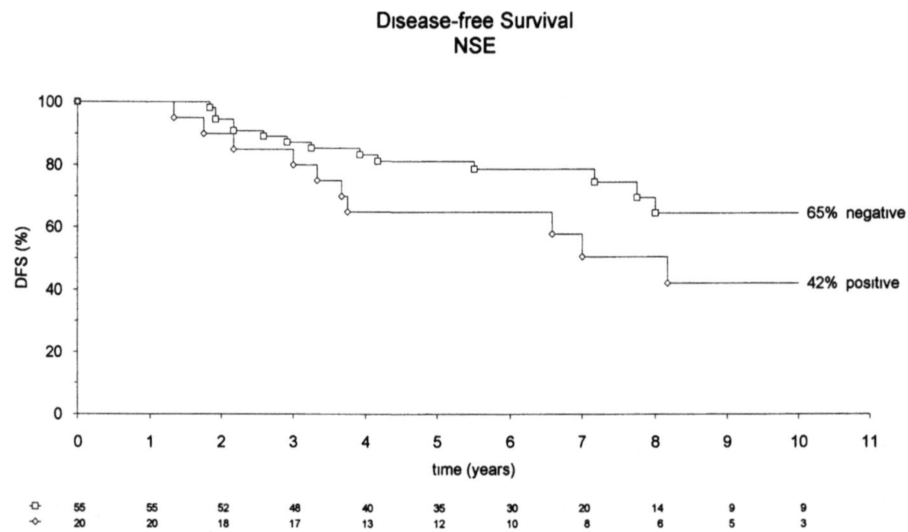

Fig. 31. Probability of disease-free survival among patients who tested positive or negative for NSE.

4.3.2 Results

Ten years after treatment, 42 % of patients whose radical prostatectomy specimen was positive for NSE and 65 % of patients whose specimen was negative for NSE were alive without evidence of disease (Figure 31). There was no statistically significant difference between the two groups of patients ($p = 0.090$). Eighty percent of patients with NSE-positive specimens and 94 % of patients with NSE-negative specimens had not died from prostate cancer after ten years (Figure 32). Again, the two groups did not differ significantly ($p = 0.160$).

For CrGrA, 75 % of patients whose specimen was positive, and 53 % of patients whose specimen was negative, were free from relapse ten years after radical prostatectomy (Figure 33). The difference between the two survival curves did not reach statistical significance ($p = 0.135$). With regard to adjusted overall survival, 100 % of CrGrA-positive and 86 % of CrGrA-negative patients had not died (Figure 34). The p-value for the difference between the two curves was 0.191 (not significant). For both NE markers, there was no association with pathological stage or histological grade.

4.3.3 Discussion

The role of neuroendocrine cells as a prognostic factor in prostate cancer is controversial. Since neuroendocrinologically differentiated tumor cells do not respond to hormonal therapy (Helpap, 1993), it has been proposed that these cells could be responsible for fatal outcome in patients with metastatic prostate cancer. Therefore, knowledge of the pre-

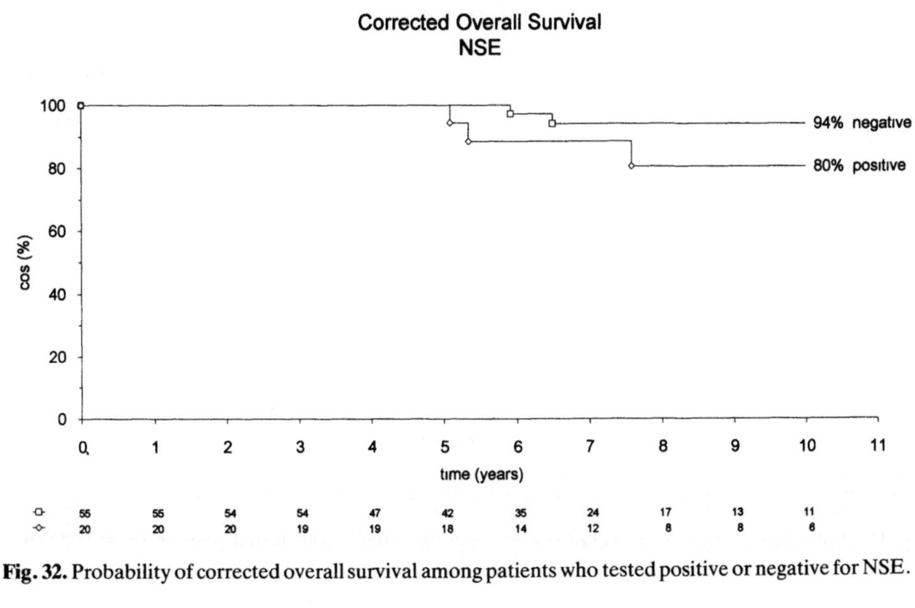

Fig. 32. Probability of corrected overall survival among patients who tested positive or negative for NSE.

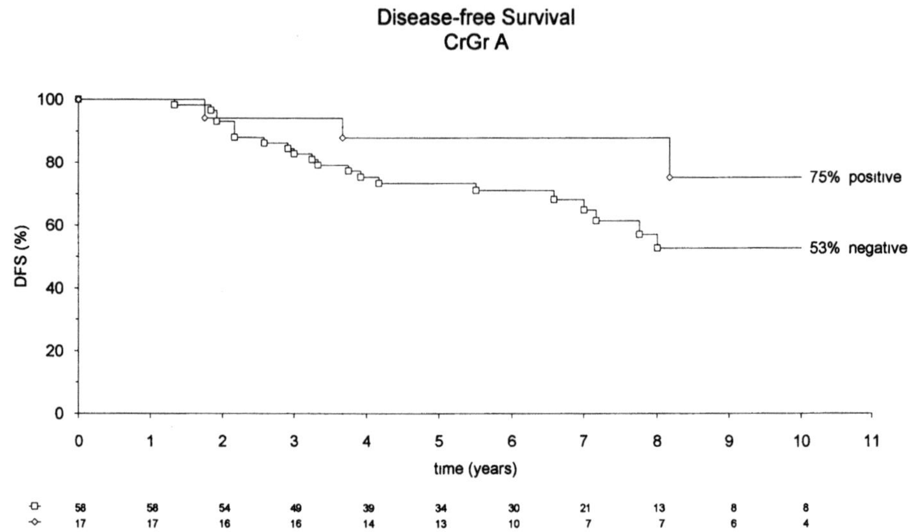

Fig. 33. Probability of disease-free survival among patients who tested positive or negative for CrGrA.

sence or absence of such NE cells might be helpful in assessing prognosis and evaluating new treatment strategies, e.g. chemotherapeutic agents, in hormone-resistant prostate cancer.

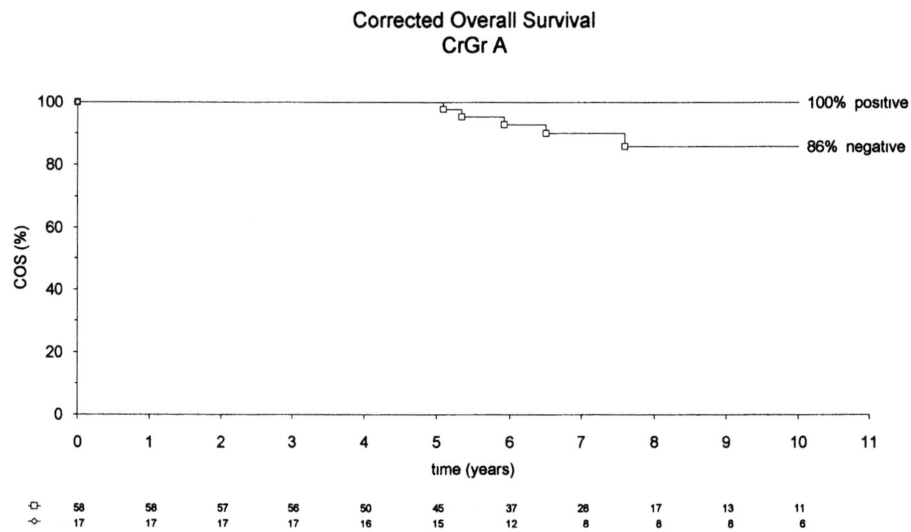

Fig. 34. Probability of corrected overall survival among patients who tested positive or negative for CrGrA.

Based on our series of radical prostatectomy treated patients, the two most commonly used markers for NE cells, NSE and CrGrA, did not have any prognostic value with regard to disease-free survival (Figures 31, 33) and corrected overall survival (Figures 32, 34), respectively. This was even the case when the dichotomous pair "positive versus negative" was gradually altered, i.e. when the extent of positivity and negativity was quantified. In no case did we find statistically significant differences between survival curves. The only other study on NE markers in radical prostatectomy came to similar results (Aprikian et al., 1993).

There are arguments for NE cells as a prognostic parameter in prostate cancer in general. Cohen et al. (1991) investigated NSE and CrGrA in 90 patients, 77 of whom were diagnosed by TURP. Radiotherapy was applied to 42 patients in clinical stages B and C; and 48 patients in stage D were primarily treated with hormones. The authors found that neuroendocrine negative tumors had a better short- and long-term prognosis than neuroendocrine positive tumors. Kadmon and colleagues (1991) measured serum CrGrA concentrations in 25 patients with disseminated prostate cancer. They found elevated CrGrA levels in 48 % of patients with stage D2, all of whom had clinical evidence of disease progression despite previous hormonal therapy. Their conclusion was that plasma CrGrA might be a marker for hormone-resistant, neuroendocrine prostate cancer cells and, thus, reflects an unfavorable prognosis.

In contrast to these reports, Tarle and Rados (1991) determined serum NSE levels in patients with untreated prostatic carcinoma. In patients with only local tumor, elevated serum NSE concentrations were found more frequently (29 %) than in subjects with disseminated disease (11 %). Aprikian et al. (1993) identified NE cells in 100 % of cases with benign prostates, in 77 % of cases with untreated prostate cancer, and in 56 % of cases with metastatic disease. They analyzed NE differentiation in radical prostatectomy specimens and found no significant differences with regard to pathological stage. Furthermore, the pattern of distribution of NE cells suggested that these cells do not retain replicative capacity. This observation was shared by Bonkhoff et al. (1991) who did not find a coexpression of the proliferation-associated Ki-67 antigen and CrGrA in the same tumor cells. Finally, the distribution of NE cells in the primary tumor did not differ from that in its metastatic deposits, implying that the metastases did not originate from NE cells (Aprikian et al., 1993).

To conclude from our study on radical prostatectomy treated patients, the two neuroendocrine markers NSE and CrGrA do not yield any prognostic information with respect to long-term follow-up.

V. References

Abrahamsson P-A, Wadstroem LB, Alumets J, Falkmer S, Grimelius L (1986) Peptide-hormone- and serotonin-immunoreactive cells in normal and hyperplastic prostate glands. Path Res Pract 181: 675

Adolfsson J, Carstensen J (1991) Natural course of clinically localized prostate adenocarcinoma in men less than 70 years old. J Urol 146: 96

Altwein JE (1982) Hormone manipulation for palliative treatment of advanced prostatic carcinoma. In: Jacobi GH, Hohenfellner R (eds): Prostate cancer. Williams & Wilkins, Baltimore-London, p. 215

Aprikian AG, Cordon-Cardo C, Fair WR, Reuter VE (1993) Characterization of neuroendocrine differentiation in human benign prostate and prostatic adenocarcinoma. Cancer 71: 3952

Bagshaw MA, Cox RS, Ray GR (1988) Status of radiation treatment of prostate cancer at Stanford University. NCI Monogr 7: 47

Beland G, Elhilali M, Fradet Y, Laroche B, Ramsey EW, Trachtenberg J, Venner PM, Tewari HD (1990) A controlled trial of castration with and without nilutamide in metastatic prostatic carcinoma. Cancer 66: 1074

Bonkhoff H, Wernert N, Dhom G, Remberger K (1991) Relation of endocrine-paracrine cells to cell proliferation in normal, hyperplastic, and neoplastic human prostate. Prostate 19: 91

Bookstein R, Allred DC (1993) Recessive oncogenes. Cancer 71: 1179

Boring CC, Squires TS, Tong T (1993) Cancer statistics, 1993. CA 43: 7

Bosch RJLH, Kurth KH, Schroeder FH (1987) Surgical treatment of locally advanced (T3) prostatic carcinoma: early results. J Urol 138: 816

Bostwick DG, Graham SD Jr, Napalkov P, Abrahamsson P-A, di Sant'Agnese PA, Algaba F, Hoisaeter PA, Lee F, Littrup P, Mostofi FK, Denis L, Schroeder F, Murphy GP (1993) Staging of early prostate cancer: a proposed tumor volume-based prognostic index. Urology 41: 403

Brawer MK (1990) Laboratory studies for the detection of carcinoma of the prostate. Urol Clin North Am 17: 759

Brawer MK (1993) The diagnosis of prostatic carcinoma. Cancer 71: 899

Breitkreuz T, Romanakis K, Lutz S, Seitz G, Bonkhoff H, Unteregger G, Zwergel T, Zang KD, Wullich B (1993) Genotypic characterization of prostatic carcinomas: a combined cytogenetic, flow cytometry, and in situ DNA hybridization study. Cancer Res 53: 4035

Burnett AL, Chan DW, Brendler CB, Walsh PC (1992) The value of serum enzymatic acid phosphatase in the staging of localized prostate cancer. J Urol 148: 1832

Cannon L, Bishop DT, Skolnick M, Hunt S, Lyon JL, Smart CR (1982) Genetic epidemiology of prostate cancer in the Utah Mormon genealogy. Cancer Surveys 1: 47

Carter BS, Beaty TH, Steinberg GD, Childs B, Walsh PC (1992a) Mendelian inheritance of familial prostate cancer. Proc Natl Acad Sci 89: 3367

Carter BS, Carter HB, Isaacs JT (1990) Epidemiologic evidence regarding predisposing factors to prostate cancer. Prostate 16: 187

Carter HB, Pearson JD, Metter EJ, Brant LJ, Chan DW, Andres R, Fozard JL, Walsh PC (1992b) Longitudinal evaluation of prostate-specific antigen levels in men with and without prostate disease. JAMA 267: 2215

Catalona WJ, Dresner SM (1985) Nerve-sparing radical prostatectomy: extraprostatic tumor extension and preservation of erectile function. J Urol 134: 1149

Catalona WJ, Smith DS, Ratliff TI, Dodds KM, Coplen DE, Yuan JJJ, Petros JA, Andriole GL (1991) Measurement of prostate-specific antigen in serum as a screening test for prostate cancer. N Engl J Med 324: 1156

Chodak GW, Bibbo M, Strauss FH II, Wied GL (1984) Transrectal aspiration biopsy versus transperineal core biopsy for the diagnosis of carcinoma of the prostate. J Urol 132: 480

Chodak GW, Keller P, Schoenberg HW (1989) Assessment of screening for prostate cancer using the digital rectal examination. J Urol 141: 1136

Chodak GW, Thisted RA, Gerber GS, Johansson J-E, Adolfsson J, Jones GW, Chisholm GD, Moskovitz B, Livne PM, Warner JW (1994) Results of conservative management of clinically localized prostate cancer. N Engl J Med 330: 242

Chybowski FM, Keller JJL, Bergstralh EJ, Oesterling JE (1991) Predicting radionuclide bone scan findings in patients with newly diagnosed, untreated prostate cancer: prostate specific antigen is superior to all other clinical parameters. J Urol 145: 313

Cohen RJ, Glezerson G, Haffejee Z (1991) Neuro-endocrine cells – a new prognostic parameter in prostate cancer. Br J Urol 68: 258

Cohen SM, Ellwein LB (1990) Cell proliferation in carcinogenesis. Science 249: 1007

Cooner WH, Mosley BR, Rutherford CL Jr, Beard JH, Pond HS, Terry WJ, Igel TC, Kidd DD (1990) Prostate cancer detection in a clinical urological practice by ultrasonography, digital rectal examination and prostate specific antigen. J Urol 143: 1146

Crawford ED, Eisenberger MA, McLeod DG, Spaulding JT, Benson R, Dorr FA, Blumenstein BA, Davis MA, Goodman PJ (1989) A controlled trial of leuprolide with and without flutamide in prostatic carcinoma. N Engl J Med 321: 419

Csapo Z, Brand K, Walther R, Fokas K (1988) Comparative experimental study of the serum prostate specific antigen and prostatic acid phosphatase in serially transplantable human prostatic carcinoma lines in nude mice. J Urol 140: 1032

Cumming JA, Ritchie AWS, Goodman CM, McIntyre MA, Chisholm GD (1990) De-differentiation with time in prostate cancer and the influence of treatment on the course of the disease. Br J Urol 65: 271

Daniels GF Jr, McNeal JE, Stamey TA (1992) Predictive value of contralateral biopsies in unilaterally palpable prostate cancer. J Urol 147: 870

de Kernion JB, Neuwirth H, Stein A, Dorey F, Stenzl A, Hannah J, Blyth B (1990) Prognosis of patients with stage D1 prostate carcinoma following radical prostatectomy with and without early endocrine therapy. J Urol 144: 700

Devesa SS, Silverman DT, Young JL Jr, Pollack ES, Brown CC, Horn JW, Percy CL, Myers MH, McKay FW, Fraumeni JF Jr (1987) Cancer incidence and mortality trends among whites in the United States, 1947-84. JNCI 79: 701

de Voogt HJ, Suciu S, Sylvester R, Pavone-Macaluso M, Smith PH, de Pauw M and Members of the European Organization for Research on Treatment of Cancer Genitourinary Tract Cancer Cooperative Group (1989) Multivariate analysis of prognostic factors in patients with advanced prostatic cancer: results from 2 european organization for research on treatment of cancer trials. J Urol 141: 883

Dhom G (1977) Classification and grading of prostatic carcinoma. In: Grundmann E, Vahlensieck W (eds): Tumors of the male genital system. Recent results in cancer research. Springer, Berlin Heidelberg New York, vol 60, p 14

di Sant'Agnese PA (1988) Neuroendocrine differentiation and prostatic carcinoma. The concept 'comes of age'. Arch Pathol Lab Med 112: 1097

di Sant'Agnese PA, de Mesy Jensen KL (1987) Neuroendocrine differentiation in prostatic carcinoma. Hum Pathol 18: 849

Donohue RE, Mani JH, Whitesel JA, Augspurger RR, Williams G, Fauver HE (1990) Intraoperative and early complications of staging pelvic lymph node dissection in prostatic adenocarcinoma. Urology 35: 223

Donohue RE, Mani JH, Whitesel JA, Mohr S, Scanavino D, Augspurger RR, Biber RJ, Fauver HE, Wettlaufer JN, Pfister RR (1982) Pelvic lymph node dissection. Guide to patient management in clinically locally confined adenocarcinoma of prostate. Urology 20: 559

Eggleston JC, Walsh PC (1985) Radical prostatectomy with preservation of sexual function: pathological results in the first 100 cases. J Urol 134: 1146

Eisbruch A, Perez CA, Roessler EH, Lockett MA (1994) Adjuvant irradiation after prostatectomy for carcinoma of the prostate with positive surgical margins. Cancer 73: 384

Eisenberger MA (1988) Chemotherapy for prostate carcinoma. NCI Monogr 7: 151

Ekman H, Hedberg K, Persson PS (1967) Cytological versus histological examination of needle biopsy specimens in the diagnosis of prostatic cancer. Br J Urol 39: 544

Elder JS, Jewett HJ, Walsh PC (1982) Radical perineal prostatectomy for clinical stage B2 carcinoma of the prostate. J Urol 127: 704
Ernster VL, Winkelstein W Jr, Selvin S, Brown SM, Sacks ST, Austin DF, Mandel SA, Bertolli TA (1977) Race, socioeconomic status, and prostate cancer. Cancer Treat Rep 61: 187
Foti AG, Herschman H, Cooper JF (1975) A solid-phase radioimmunoassay for human prostatic acid phosphatase. Cancer Res 35: 2446
Foulds L (1954) The experimental study of tumor progression: a review. Cancer Res 14: 327
Foulds L (1958) The natural history of cancer. J Chronic Dis 8: 2
Franks LM (1954) Latent carcinoma of the prostate. J Pathol Bacteriol 68: 603
Franks LM (1956) Latency and progression in tumours: The natural history of prostatic cancer. Lancet 2: 1037
Franzen S, Giertz G, Zajicek J (1960) Cytological diagnosis of prostatic tumours by transrectal aspiration biopsy: a preliminary report. Br J Urol 32: 193
Freiha FS, Bagshaw MA (1984) Carcinoma of the prostate: results of post-irradiation biopsy. Prostate 5: 19
Friedman GD, Hiatt RA, Quesenberry CP Jr, Selby JV (1991) Case-control study of screening for prostatic cancer by digital rectal examinations. Lancet 337: 1526
Frohmueller H, Wirth M, Manseck A, Theiss M (1991) Selektionskriterien fuer die radikale Prostatektomie unter Beruecksichtigung von Langzeitergebnissen. Urologe [A] 30: 394
George NJR (1988) Natural history of localised prostatic cancer managed by conservative therapy alone. Lancet I: 494
Gervasi LA, Mata J, Easley JD, Wilbanks JH, Seale-Hawkins C, Carlton CE Jr, Scardino PT (1989) Prognostic significance of lymph nodal metastases in prostate cancer. J Urol 142: 332
Gibbons RP, Correa RJ Jr, Brannen GE, Mason JT (1984) Total prostatectomy for localized prostatic cancer. J Urol 131: 73
Giovannucci E, Ascherio A, Rimm EB, Colditz GA, Stampfer MJ, Willett WC (1993a) A prospective cohort study of vasectomy and prostate cancer in US men. JAMA 269: 873
Giovannucci E, Tosteson TD, Speizer FE, Ascherio A, Vessey MP, Colditz GA (1993b) A retrospective cohort study of vasectomy and prostate cancer in US men. JAMA 269: 878
Gleason DF (1977) Histologic grading and clinical staging of prostatic carcinoma. In: Tannenbaum M (ed): Urologic Pathology: the prostate. Philadelphia, Lea & Febiger, p. 171
Gleason DF, Mellinger GT, and the VACURG (1974) Prediction of prognosis for prostatic adenocarcinoma by combined histological grading and clinical staging. J Urol 111: 58
Goldie JH (1987) Scientific basis for adjuvant and primary (neoadjuvant) chemotherapy. Semin Oncol 14: 1
Goldie JH, Coldman AJ (1979) A mathematic model for relating the drug sensitivity of tumors to their spontaneous mutation rate. Cancer Treat Rep 63: 1727
Graves HCB, Kamarei M, Stamey TA (1990a) Identity of prostate specific antigen and the semen protein p30 purified by a rapid chromatography technique. J Urol 144: 1510
Graves HCB, Wehner N, Stamey TA (1990b) Comparison of a polyclonal and monoclonal immunoassay for PSA: need for an international antigen standard. J Urol 144: 1516
Guileyardo JM, Johnson WD, Welsh RA, Akazaki K, Correa P (1980) Prevalence of latent prostate carcinoma in two U.S. populations. JNCI 65: 311
Gutman AB, Gutman EB (1938) An "acid" phosphatase occuring in the serum of patients with metastasizing carcinoma of the prostate gland. J Clin Invest 17: 473
Haeggman M, Norberg M, de la Torre M, Fritjofsson A, Busch C (1993) Characterization of localized prostatic cancer: distribution, grading and pT-staging in radical prostatectomy specimens. Scand J Urol Nephrol 27: 7
Hall GS, Kramer CE, Epstein JI (1991) Partial sampling methods of radical prostatectomy specimens. J Urol 145: 253A
Hammerer P, Huland H (1991) Zur Diagnostik des lokalisierten Prostatakarzinoms: Screening und praeoperatives Staging. Urologe [A] 30: 378
Hammerer P, Huland H (1994) Systematic sextant biopsies in 651 patients referred for prostate evaluation. J Urol 151: 99
Hammerer P, Huland H, Sparenberg A (1992) Digital rectal examination, imaging, and systematic-sextant biopsy in identifying operable lymph node-negative prostatic carcinoma. Eur Urol 22: 281
Hanahan D (1989) Transgenic mice as probes into complex systems. Science 246: 1265

Heller JE (1987) Prostatic acid phosphatase: its current clinical status. J Urol 137: 1091
Helpap B (1993) Future directions in research of prostate carcinoma. Path Res Pract 189: 497
Helpap B (1989) Pathologie der ableitenden Harnwege und der Prostata. Springer, Berlin Heidelberg New York
Herbst RH, Polkey HJ (1933) Prostatic malignancy. In: Ballenger EG, Frontz WA, Hamer HG (eds): History of Urology, Vol II, Williams & Wilkins, Baltimore, p. 187
Hering F, Mueller S (1991) 31-P MR spectroscopy and 1-H MR imaging of the human prostate using a transrectal probe. Urol Res 19: 349
Hering F, Rist M, Roth J, Mihatsch M, Rutishauser G (1990) Does microinvasion of the capsule and/or micrometastases in regional lymph nodes influence disease-free survival after radical prostatectomy? Br J Urol 66: 177
Hermanek P, Sobin LH (eds) (1987) TNM classification of malignant tumours. In: International Union against Cancer. Springer, Berlin Heidelberg New York
Hodge KK, McNeal JE, Stamey TA (1989a) Ultrasound guided transrectal core biopsies of the palpably abnormal prostate. J Urol 142: 66
Hodge KK, McNeal JE, Terris MK, Stamey TA (1989b) Random systematic versus directed ultrasound guided transrectal core biopsies of the prostate. J Urol 142: 71
Horm JW, Sondik EJ (1989) Person-years of life lost due to cancer in the United States, 1970 and 1984. Am J Public Health 79: 1490
Hsu S-E, Raine L, Fanger H (1981) Use of avidin-biotin-peroxidase complex (ABC) in immunoperoxidase techniques: a comparison between ABC and unlabeled antibody (PAP) procedures. J Histochem Cytochem 29: 577
Huber PR, Hering F, Rist M, Misteli R, Rutishauser G (1986) Prostate specific antigen (PSA): experimental and clinical data. Urol Res 14: 164
Huber PR, Schnell Y, Hering F, Rutishauser G (1987) Prostate specific antigen. Experimental and clinical observations. Scand J Urol Nephrol 104: 33
Huber PR, Scholer A, Linder E, Hagmaier V, Vogt H, Christen P, Eppenberger U, Rutishauser G (1982) Measurement of prostatic acid phosphatase in serum and bone marrow: radioimmunoassay and enzymatic measurement compared. Clin Chem 28: 2044
Huggins C, Hodges CV (1941) Studies on prostatic cancer. I. The effect of castration, of estrogen and of androgen injection on serum phosphatases in metastatic carcinoma of the prostate. Cancer Res 1: 293
Humphrey PA, Vollmer RT (1990) Intraglandular tumor extent and prognosis in prostatic carcinoma: application of a grid method to prostatectomy specimens. Hum Pathol 21: 799
Janknegt RA, Abbou CC, Bartoletti R, Bernstein-Hahn L, Bracken B, Brisset JM, Calais da Silva F, Chisholm G, Crawford ED, Debruyne FMJ, Dijkman GD, Frick J, Goedhals L, Knoenagel H, Venner PM (1993) Orchiectomy and nilutamide or placebo as treatment of metastatic prostatic cancer in a multinational double-blind randomized trial. J Urol 149: 77
Jewett HJ (1956) Significance of the palpable prostatic nodule. JAMA 160: 838
Jewett HJ (1975) The present status of radical prostatectomy for stages A and B prostatic cancer. Urol Clin North Am 2: 105
Jewett HJ (1980) Radical perineal prostatectomy for palpable, clinically localized, non-obstructive cancer: experience at the Johns Hopkins Hospital 1909-1963. J Urol 124: 492
Jewett HJ, Eggleston JC, Yawn DH (1972) Radical prostatectomy in the management of carcinoma of the prostate: probable causes of some therapeutic failures. J Urol 107: 1034
Johansson J-E, Adami H-O, Andersson S-O, Bergstroem R, Holmberg L, Krusemo UB (1992a) High 10-year survival rate in patients with early, untreated prostatic cancer. JAMA 267: 2191
Johansson J-E, Adami H-O, Andersson S-O, Bergstroem R, Krusemo UB, Kraaz W (1989) Natural history of localised prostatic cancer. A population-based study in 223 untreated patients. Lancet I: 799
Johansson J-E, Sigurdsson T, Holmberg L, Bergstroem R (1992b) Erythrocyte sedimentation rate as a tumor marker in human prostatic cancer. An analysis of prognostic factors in 300 population-based consecutive cases. Cancer 70: 1556
Kabalin JN, Hodge KK, McNeal JE, Freiha FS, Stamey TA (1989) Identification of residual cancer in the prostate following radiation therapy: role of transrectal ultrasound guided biopsy and prostate specific antigen. J Urol 142: 326
Kadmon D, Thompson TC, Lynch GR, Scardino PT (1991) Elevated plasma chromogranin-A concentrations in prostatic carcinoma. J Urol 146: 358

Kaplan EL, Meier P (1958) Nonparametric estimation from incomplete observations. J Am Stat Assoc 53: 457

Kaplan ID, Bagshaw MA (1992) Serum prostate-specific antigen after post-prostatectomy radiotherapy. Urology 39: 401

Kastendieck H (1984) Klassifikation, Morphologie und Pathogenese des inzidenten Prostatakarzinoms. In: Helpap B, Senge T, Vahlensieck W (Hrsg): Die Prostata. Band 2. pmi, Frankfurt, S. 133

Kavoussi LR, Sosa E, Chandhoke P, Chodak G, Clayman RV, Hadley HR, Loughlin KR, Ruckle HC, Rukstalis D, Schuessler W, Segura J, Vancaille T, Winfield HN (1993) Complications of laparoscopic pelvic lymph node dissection. J Urol 149: 322

Kennedy TJ, Sonneland AM, Marlett MM, Troup RH (1992) Luteinizing hormone-releasing hormone downstaging of clinical stage C prostate cancer. J Urol 147: 891

Knoenagel H, Hauri D (1984) Prostatadiagnostik – genuegt die Zytologie? Helv chir Acta 51: 433

Kozlowski JM, Ellis WJ, Grayhack JT (1991) Advanced prostatic carcinoma: Early versus late endocrine therapy. Urol Clin North Am 18: 15

Kuechler HK (1866) Ueber Prostatavergroesserungen, Deutsche Klinik. Zeitschrift fuer Beobachtungen aus deutschen Kliniken und Krankenhaeusern. Reimer, Berlin

Labrie F, Dupont A, Belanger A, Lacoursiere Y, Raynaud JP, Husson JM, Gareau J, Fazekas ATA, Sandow J, Monfette G, Girard JG, Emond J, Houle JG (1983) New approach in the treatment of prostate cancer: complete instead of partial withdrawal of androgens. Prostate 4: 579

Lange PH, Lightner DJ, Medini E, Reddy PK, Vessella RL (1990) The effect of radiation therapy after radical prostatectomy in patients with elevated prostate specific antigen levels. J Urol 144: 927

Lange PH, Narayan P (1983) Understaging and undergrading of prostate cancer. Argument for post-operative radiation as adjuvant therapy. Urology 21: 113

Lee F, Torp-Pedersen S, Littrup PJ, McLeary RD, McHugh TA, Smid AP, Stella PJ, Borlaza GS (1989) Hypoechoic lesions of the prostate: clinical relevance of tumor size, digital rectal examination, and prostate-specific antigen. Radiology 170: 29

Lew EA, Garfinkel L (1990) Mortality at ages 75 and older in the Cancer Prevention Study (CPSI). CA 40: 210

Linehan WM, LaRocca R, Stein C, Walther M, Cooper M, Weiss G, Choyke P, Cassidy J, Uhrich M, Myers CE (1990) Use of suramin in treatment of patients with advanced prostate carcinoma. J Urol 143: 221A

Link P, Freiha FS, Stamey TA (1991) Adjuvant radiation therapy in patients with detectable prostate specific antigen following radical prostatectomy. J Urol 145: 532

Lloyd RV, Wilson BS (1983) Specific endocrine tissue marker defined by a monoclonal antibody. Science 222: 628

Lowe BA, Listrom MB (1988) Incidental carcinoma of the prostate: an analysis of the predictors of progression. J Urol 140: 1340

Macfarlane MT, Abi-Aad A, Stein A, Danella J, Belldegrun A, deKernion JB (1993) Neoadjuvant hormonal deprivation in patients with locally advanced prostate cancer. J Urol 150: 132

Madsen PO, Graversen PH, Gasser TC, Corle DK (1988) Treatment of localized prostatic cancer. Radical prostatectomy versus placebo. A 15-year follow-up. Scand J Urol Nephrol 110: 95

Mantel N (1966) Evaluation of survival data and two new rank order statistics arising in its consideration. Cancer Chemother Rep 50: 163

McCullough DK, Leadbetter WF (1972) Radical pelvic surgery for locally extensive carcinoma of the prostate. J Urol 108: 939

McNeal JE (1969) Origin and development of carcinoma in the prostate. Cancer 23: 24

McNeal JE, Bostwick DG, Kindrachuk RA, Redwine EA, Freiha FS, Stamey TA (1986) Patterns of progression in prostate cancer. Lancet 1: 60

McNeal JE, Price HM, Redwine EA, Freiha FS, Stamey TA (1988) Stage A versus Stage B adenocarcinoma of the prostate: morphological comparison and biological significance. J Urol 139: 61

McNeal JE, Villers AA, Redwine EA, Freiha FS, Stamey TA (1990a) Capsular penetration in prostate cancer. Significance for natural history and treatment. Am J Surg Pathol 14: 240

McNeal JE, Villers AA, Redwine EA, Freiha FS, Stamey TA (1990b) Histologic differentiation, cancer volume, and pelvic lymph node metastasis in adenocarcinoma of the prostate. Cancer 66: 1225

Meyer JS, Sufrin G, Martin SA (1982) Proliferative activity of benign human prostate, prostatic adenocarcinoma and seminal vesicle evaluated by thymidine labeling. J Urol 128: 1353

Mihatsch MJ (1994) Personal communication
Millin T (1945) Retropubic prostatectomy. A new extravesical technique. Report on 20 cases. Lancet 2: 693
Montie JE, Wood DP Jr, Pontes JE, Boyett JM, Levin HS (1989) Adenocarcinoma of the prostate in cystoprostatectomy specimens removed for bladder cancer. Cancer 63: 381
Moul JW, Paulson DF (1991) The role of radical surgery in the management of radiation recurrent and large volume prostate cancer. Cancer 68: 1265
Mueller H-A, Altenaehr E, Boecking A, Dhom G, Faul P, Goettinger H, Helpap B, Hohbach C, Kastendieck H, Leistenschneider W (1980) Ueber Klassifikation und Grading des Prostatakarzinoms. Verh Dtsch Ges Pathol 64: 609
Mukamel E, deKernion JB, Dorey F, Hannah J (1990) Significance of histological prognostic indicators in patients with carcinoma of the prostate. Br J Urol 65: 46
Mukamel E, Hannah J, Barbaric Z, deKernion JB (1986) The value of computerized tomography scan and magnetic resonance imaging in staging prostatic carcinoma: comparison with the clinical and histological staging. J Urol 136: 1231
Murphy LJT (1972) The history of Urology. Charles C Thomas, Springfield, Illinois, USA
National Center for Health Statistics (1986) Vital statistics of the United States. Hyattsville, MD: Public Health Service 2: 10
National Institutes of Health consensus development conference, June 15-17, 1987 (1987) The management of clinically localized prostate cancer. J Urol 138: 1369
Nemoto R, Uchida K, Shimazui T, Hattori K, Koiso K, Harada M (1989) Immunocytochemical demonstration of S phase cells by anti-bromodeoxyuridine monoclonal antibody in human prostate adenocarcinoma. J Urol 141: 337
Nicolson GL (1987) Tumor cell instability, diversification, and progression to the metastatic phenotype: from oncogene to oncofetal expression. Cancer Res 47: 1473
Nienhuis H, Goldacre M, Seagroatt V, Gill L, Vessey M (1992) Incidence of disease after vasectomy: a record linkage retrospective cohort study. BMJ 304: 743
Noble RL (1977) The development of prostatic adenocarcinoma in Nb rats following prolonged sex hormone administration. Cancer Res 37: 1929
Nseyo UO, Pontes JE (1989) Intraprostatic tumor location and pelvic lymph node metastatic pattern in early prostate cancer. Urology 33: 171
Oesterling JE (1991) Prostate-specific antigen: a critical assessment of the most useful tumor marker for adenocarcinoma of the prostate. J Urol 145: 907
Oesterling JE, Andrews PE, Suman VJ, Zincke H, Myers RP (1993) Preoperative androgen deprivation therapy: artificial lowering of serum prostate specific antigen without downstaging the tumor. J Urol 149: 779
Oesterling JE, Chan DW, Epstein JI, Kimball AW Jr, Bruzek DJ, Rock RC, Brendler CB, Walsh PC (1988) Prostate specific antigen in the preoperative and postoperative evaluation of localized prostatic cancer treated with radical prostatectomy. J Urol 139: 766
Palken M, Cobb OE, Warren BH, Hoak DC (1990) Prostate cancer: correlation of digital rectal examination, transrectal ultrasound and prostate specific antigen levels with tumor volumes in radical prostatectomy specimens. J Urol 143: 1155
Partin AW, Borland RN, Epstein JI, Brendler CB (1993) Influence of wide excision of the neurovascular bundle(s) on prognosis in men with clinically localized prostate cancer with established capsular penetration. J Urol 150: 142
Partin AW, Carter HB, Chan DW, Epstein JI, Oesterling JE, Rock RC, Weber JP, Walsh PC (1990) Prostate specific antigen in the staging of localized prostate cancer: influence of tumor differentiation, tumor volume and benign hyperplasia. J Urol 143: 747
Partin AW, Epstein JI, Cho KR, Gittelsohn AM, Walsh PC (1989) Morphometric measurement of tumor volume and per cent of gland involvement as predictors of pathological stage in clinical stage B prostate cancer. J Urol 141: 341
Paulson DF, Hodge GB Jr, Hinshaw W and the Uro-Oncology Research Group (1984) Radiation therapy versus delayed androgen deprivation for stage C carcinoma of the prostate. J Urol 131: 901
Paulson DF, Lin GH, Hinshaw W, Stephani S and the Uro-Oncology Research Group (1982) Radical surgery versus radiotherapy for adenocarcinoma of the prostate. J Urol 128: 502
Paulson DF, Moul JW, Walther PJ (1990) Radical prostatectomy for clinical stage T1-2N0M0 prostatic adenocarcinoma: long-term results. J Urol 144: 1180

Peehl DM (1993) Oncogenes in prostate cancer. An update. Cancer 71: 1159
Peehl DM, Wong ST, Stamey TA (1991) Cytostatic effects of suramin on prostate cancer cells cultured from primary tumors. J Urol 145: 624
Perrin P, Francois O, Maquet JH, Bringeon G, Duteil P, Devonec M (1991) Circulating prostate-specific antigen in benign hypertrophy and localized cancer of the prostate: can PSA be considered as a screening examination for localized cancer? Progres en Urol 1: 419
Petros JA, Catalona WJ (1992) Lower incidence of unsuspected lymph node metastases in 521 consecutive patients with clinically localized prostate cancer. J Urol 147: 1574
Quinlan DM, Epstein JI, Carter BS, Walsh PC (1991) Sexual function following radical prostatectomy: influence of preservation of neurovascular bundles. J Urol 145: 998
Ragde H, Aldape HC, Bagley CM Jr (1988) Ultrasound-guided prostate biopsy. Biopty gun superior to aspiration. Urology 32: 503
Rich AR (1935) On the frequency of occurence of occult carcinoma of the prostate. J Urol 33: 215
Rifkin MD, Zerhouni EA, Gatsonis CA, Quint LE, Paushter DM, Epstein JI, Hamper U, Walsh PC, McNeil BJ (1990) Comparison of magnetic resoncance imaging and ultrasonography in staging early prostate cancer. Results of a multi-institutional cooperative trial. N Engl J Med 323: 621
Ritter MA, Messing EM, Shanahan TG, Potts S, Chappell RJ, Kinsella TJ (1992) Prostate-specific antigen as a predictor of radiotherapy response and patterns of failure in localized prostate cancer. J Clin Oncol 10: 1208
Rodin AE, Larson DL, Roberts DK (1967) Nature of the perineural space invaded by prostatic carcinoma. Cancer 20: 1772
Roy AV, Brower ME, Hayden JE (1971) Sodium thymolphthalein monophosphate: a new acid phosphatase substrate with greater specificity for the prostatic enzyme in serum. Clin Chem 17: 1093
Ruebben H, Altwein JE (1987) Das fortgeschrittene Prostatakarzinom – Ein therapeutisches Dilemma? Urologe [A] 26: 7
Sager R (1989) Tumor suppressor genes: the puzzle and the promise. Science 246: 1406
Sarosdy MF (1990) Do we have a rational treatment plan for stage D-1 carcinoma of the prostate? World J Urol 8: 27
Sassine AM, Schulman C (1993) Clinical use of prostate-specific antigen in staging of patients with prostatic carcinoma. Eur Urol 23: 348
Scardino PT (1989) Early detection of prostate cancer. Urol Clin North Am 16: 635
Schaffer DL, Pendergrass HP (1976) Comparison of enzyme, clinical, radiographic, and radionuclide methods of detecting bone metastases from carcinoma of the prostate. Radiology 121: 431
Schellhammer PF, El-Mahdi AM, Higgins EM, Schultheiss TE, Ladaga LE, Babb TJ (1987) Prostate biopsy after definitive treatment by interstitial 125-Iodine implant or external beam radiation therapy. J Urol 137: 897
Schmassmann A, Mihatsch MJ (1983) Das Prostatakarzinom. Die Haeufigkeit und Bedeutung des „Stadiums I" – praeklinisches Karzinom. Urologe [A] 22: 388
Schmid H-P (1991) The problem of obstruction in prostate cancer. Urol Res 19: 323
Schmid H-P, McNeal JE (1992) An abbreviated standard procedure for accurate tumor volume estimation in prostate cancer. Am J Surg Pathol 16: 184
Schmid H-P, McNeal JE, Stamey TA (1993) Observations on the doubling time of prostate cancer. The use of serial prostate-specific antigen in patients with untreated disease as a measure of increasing cancer volume. Cancer 71: 2031
Schmid H-P, Stamey TA, McNeal JE, Freiha FS, Redwine EA, Whittemore AS (1994) Einfluss der natuerlichen Geschichte auf die Handhabung des Adenokarzinoms der Prostata. Urologe [A] 33: 144
Schnall MD, Lenkinski RE, Pollack HM, Imai Y, Kressel HY (1989) Prostate: MR imaging with an endorectal surface coil. Radiology 127: 570
Schroeder FH (1991) Radikale Prostatektomie und adjuvante endokrine Behandlung beim lymphogen metastasierten Prostatakarzinom? Urologe [A] 30: 417
Scott WW, Boyd HL (1969) Combined hormone control therapy and radical prostatectomy in the treatment of selected cases of advanced carcinoma of the prostate: a retrospective study based upon 25 years of experience. J Urol 101: 86
Sensabaugh GF (1978) Isolation and characterization of a semen specific protein from human seminal plasma: a potential new marker for semen identification. J Forensic Sci 23: 106

Shackney SE, McCormack GW, Cuchural GJ Jr (1978) Growth rate patterns of solid tumors and their relation to responsiveness to therapy. An analytical review. Ann Intern Med 89: 107

Skowronski RJ, Peehl DM, Feldman D (1993) Vitamin D and prostate cancer: 1,25 dihydroxyvitamin D3 receptors and actions in human prostate cancer cell lines. Endocrinology 132: 1952

Smith JA Jr, Middleton RG (1985) Implications of volume of nodal metastasis in patients with adenocarcinoma of the prostate. J Urol 133: 617

Smith JA Jr, Seaman JP, Gleidman JB, Middleton RG (1983) Pelvic lymph node metastasis from prostatic cancer: influence of tumor grade and stage in 452 consecutive patients. J Urol 130: 290

Smith PH (1991) Quality of survival in metastatic prostatic cancer. Rev on endocrine-rel cancer 37: 15

Spigelman SS, McNeal JE, Freiha FS, Stamey TA (1986) Rectal examination in volume determination of carcinoma of the prostate: clinical and anatomical correlations. J Urol 136: 1228

Spitz MR, Currier RD, Fueger JJ, Babaian RJ, Newell GR (1991) Familial patterns of prostate cancer: a case-control analysis. J Urol 146: 1305

Spratt JS, Heuser L, Kuhns JG, Reiman HM, Buchanan JB, Polk HC Jr, Sandoz J (1981) Association between the actual doubling times of primary breast cancer with histopathologic characteristics and Wolfe's parenchymal mammographic patterns. Cancer 47: 2265

Stamey TA, Dietrick DD, Issa MM (1993a) Large, organ confined, impalpable transition zone prostate cancer: association with metastatic levels of prostate specific antigen. J Urol 149: 510

Stamey TA, Ferrari MK, Schmid H-P (1993b) The value of serial prostate specific antigen determinations 5 years after radiotherapy: steeply increasing values characterize 80 % of patients. J Urol 150: 1856

Stamey TA, Freiha FS, McNeal JE, Redwine EA, Whittemore AS, Schmid H-P (1993c) Localized prostate cancer. Relationship of tumor volume to clinical significance for treatment of prostate cancer. Cancer 71: 933

Stamey TA, Kabalin JN (1989) Prostate specific antigen in the diagnosis and treatment of adenocarcinoma of the prostate. I. untreated patients. J Urol 141: 1070

Stamey TA, Kabalin JN, McNeal JE, Johnston IM, Freiha FS, Redwine EA, Yang N (1989) Prostate specific antigen in the diagnosis and treatment of adenocarcinoma of the prostate. II. radical prostatectomy treated patients. J Urol 141: 1076

Stamey TA, McNeal JE (1992) Adenocarcinoma of the prostate. In: Campbell's Urology, 6th Edition. Edited by PC Walsh, AB Retik, TA Stamey and ED Vaughan Jr. Philadelphia: WB Saunders, vol 2, chap 29, p 1159

Stamey TA, McNeal JE, Freiha FS, Rewine E (1988) Morphometric and clinical studies on 68 consecutive radical prostatectomies. J Urol 139: 1235

Stamey TA, Yang N, Hay AR, McNeal JE, Freiha FS, Redwine E (1987) Prostate-specific antigen as a serum marker for adenocarcinoma of the prostate. N Engl J Med 317: 909

Stein A, deKernion JB, Dorey F, Smith RB (1992) Adjuvant radiotherapy in patients post-radical prostatectomy with tumor extending through capsule or positive seminal vesicles. Urology 39: 59

Steinberg GD, Carter BS, Beaty TH, Childs B, Walsh PC (1990a) Family history and the risk of prostate cancer. Prostate 17: 337

Steinberg GD, Epstein JI, Piantadosi S, Walsh PC (1990b) Management of stage D1 adenocarcinoma of the prostate: the Johns Hopkins experience 1974 to 1987. J Urol 144: 1425

Stenzl A, Studer UE (1993) Outcome of patients with untreated cancer of the prostate. Eur Urol 24: 1

Stilmant MM, Freelund MC, de las Morenas A, Shepard RL, Oates RD, Siroky MB (1989) Expanded role for fine needle aspiration of the prostate. A study of 335 specimens. Cancer 63: 583

Surveillance, Epidemiology, and End Results (1981) Incidence and mortality data: 1973-1977. Bethesda (MD): National Cancer Institute Monogr 57; Publication No. (NIH) 81-2330

Tarle M, Rados N (1991) Investigation on serum neurone-specific enolase in prostate cancer diagnosis and monitoring: comparative study of a multiple tumor marker assay. Prostate 19: 23

Terris MK, McNeal JE, Stamey TA (1992) Transrectal ultrasound imaging and ultrasound guided prostate biopsies in the detection of residual carcinoma in clinical stage A carcinoma of the prostate. J Urol 147: 864

Tyrrell CJ, Altwein JE, Klippel F, Varenhorst E, Lunglmayr G, Boccardo F, Holdaway IM, Haefliger J-M, Jordaan JP and Sotarauta M for the International Prostate Cancer Study Group (1991) A multicenter randomized trial comparing the luteinizing hormone-releasing hormone analogue goserelin acetate alone and with flutamide in the treatment of advanced prostate cancer. J Urol 146: 1321

Van den Ouden D, Boeve E, Schroeder FH (1992) The importance of the capsular penetration state in radical prostatectomy specimens of patients with a prostatic carcinoma. Impact on time to progression. J Urol 147: 304A

Veterans Administration Co-operative Urological Research Group (1967a) Treatment and survival of patients with cancer of the prostate. Surg Gynecol Obstet 124: 1011

Veterans Administration Cooperative Urological Research Group (1967b) Carcinoma of the prostate: treatment comparisons. J Urol 98: 516

Villers A, McNeal JE, Freiha FS, Boccon-Gibod L, Stamey TA (1993) Invasion of Denonvillier's fascia in radical prostatectomy specimens. J Urol 149: 793

Villers A, McNeal JE, Redwine EA, Freiha FS, Stamey TA (1989) The role of perineural space invasion in the local spread of prostatic adenocarcinoma. J Urol 142: 763

Villers AA, McNeal JE, Redwine EA, Freiha FS, Stamey TA (1990) Pathogenesis and biological significance of seminal vesicle invasion in prostatic adenocarcinoma. J Urol 143: 1183

Viola MV, Fromowitz F, Oravez S, Deb S, Finkel G, Lundy J, Hand P, Thor A, Schlom J (1986) Expression of ras oncogene p21 in prostate cancer. N Engl J Med 314: 133

Voges G, Hohenfellner R (1990) Prostatakarzinom: Keine Behandlung – eine Option bei klinisch lokalisiertem Tumor? Akt Urol 21: 232

Voges GE, McNeal JE, Redwine EA, Freiha FS, Stamey TA (1992a) Morphologic analysis of surgical margins with positive findings in prostatectomy for adenocarcinoma of the prostate. Cancer 69: 520

Voges GE, McNeal JE, Redwine EA, Freiha FS, Stamey TA (1992b) The predictive significance of substaging stage A prostate cancer (A1 versus A2) for volume and grade of total cancer in the prostate. J Urol 147: 858

Walsh PC, Donker PJ (1982) Impotence following radical prostatectomy: insight into etiology and prevention. J Urol 128: 492

Walsh PC, Lepor H, Eggleston JC (1983) Radical prostatectomy with preservation of sexual function: anatomical and pathological considerations. Prostate 4: 473

Wang MC, Valenzuela LA, Murphy GP, Chu TM (1979) Purification of a human prostate specific antigen. Invest Urol 17: 159

Watanabe H, Igari D, Tanahashi Y, Harada K, Saitoh M (1975) Transrectal ultrasonotomography of the prostate. J Urol 114: 734

Wheeler TM (1989) Anatomic considerations in carcinoma of the prostate. Urol Clin North Am 16: 623

Whitmore WF Jr (1956) Hormone therapy in prostatic cancer. Am J Med 21: 697

Whitmore WF Jr (1973) The natural history of prostatic cancer. Cancer 32: 1104

Whitmore WF Jr (1988) Overview: historical and contemporary. NCI Monogr 7: 7

Whitmore WF Jr, Warner JA, Thompson IM Jr (1991) Expectant management of localized prostatic cancer. Cancer 67: 1091

Wirth MP, Frohmueller HGW (1992) Prostate-specific antigen and prostate acid phosphatase in the detection of early prostate cancer and the prediction of regional lymph node metastases. Eur Urol 22: 27

Woolf CM (1960) An investigation of the familial aspects of carcinoma of the prostate. Cancer 13: 739

Young HH (1905) The early diagnosis and radical cure of carcinoma of the prostate. Being a study of 40 cases and presentation of a radical operation which was carried out in four cases. Bull Johns Hopkins Hosp 16: 315

Zaridze DG, Boyle P (1987) Cancer of the prostate: epidemiology and aetiology. Br J Urol 59: 493

Ziegler M, Mast G, Becht E, Moll V (1990) Radical prostatectomy versus high voltage radiotherapy in treatment of the locoregional prostatic carcinoma. Akt Urol 21: 25

Zincke H (1989) Extended experience with surgical treatment of stage D1 adenocarcinoma of prostate. Significant influences of immediate adjuvant hormonal treatment (orchiectomy) on outcome. Urology 33: 27

Zincke H, Utz DC, Taylor WF (1986) Bilateral pelvic lymphadenectomy and radical prostatectomy for clinical stage C prostatic cancer: role of adjuvant treatment for residual cancer and in disease progression. J Urol 135: 1199

VI. Summary

Adenocarcinoma of the prostate is the most common of all male cancers in Western countries except for skin cancer and second only to lung cancer in mortality. Through the introduction of prostate-specific antigen (PSA) and transrectal ultrasonography with biopsy a few years ago, more and more prostate cancers have been diagnosed. However, the discrepancy between histologically identifiable carcinomas (40 % in autopsy series and in cystoprostatectomy series for bladder cancer, respectively) and clinically diagnosed carcinomas (8 % probability for a man being diagnosed within his entire life) has led to a considerable diagnostic and therapeutic dilemma. Prostate cancer was said to have an unpredictable natural course and selection criteria for radical prostatectomy and prognostic parameters in view of long-term follow-up were not well defined. The present monograph consists of four parts: a review on prostatic cancer in general, clinical studies on the natural history, clinical studies on selection criteria for curative surgery, and morphological and immunohistochemical investigations on various prognostic factors in radical prostatectomy specimens.

In the first chapter, a brief overview on historical, epidemiological and etiological aspects is given. Current diagnostic approaches and different treatment modalities are discussed.

The second part on the natural history is based on previous work from the Stanford group. The biological aggressiveness of prostate cancer (capsular penetration, seminal vesicle invasion, pelvic lymph node metastasis) is directly related to tumor volume and quantitated histological grade. In a further study based on the proportional relationship between tumor volume and serum PSA, untreated patients with prostate cancer were followed by serial PSA determinations. It could be demonstrated that the increase of serum PSA is exponential over time in all clinical stages and that median doubling time for clinically organ-confined tumors is four years. This extraordinary slow growth rate (doubling time) of prostate cancer has substantial consequences for early diagnosis and therapeutic management.

In section three, preoperative (clinical) selection criteria for prediction of pathologically organ-confined disease were evaluated in our Basel series of 140 consecutive radical prostatectomies. It was found that serum PSA is superior to both digital rectal examination and prostatic acid phosphatase. In patients with a PSA in the normal range (up to 12 ng/ml by the polyclonal Yang assay), a staging lymphadenectomy can be omitted because these low volume cancers do not show positive nodes.

In the fourth chapter, two abbreviated standard procedures for accurate tumor volume estimation in radical prostatectomy specimens are described. They have been validated in 145 cases from the original Stanford method. Furthermore, in our Basel series with a mean follow-up of eight years, pathological stage and seminal vesicle involvement are strong prognostic parameters with regard to disease-free survival and corrected overall survival. Minimal pelvic lymph node metastasis (pN1.1) does not influence outcome. The neuroendocrine markers neuron-specific enolase and chromogranin-A were found to have no prognostic significance.

VII. Acknowledgments

I would like to thank Prof. Georg Rutishauser, without whose support this thesis would not have been possible.

I am very grateful to Prof. Thomas A. Stamey and Prof. John E. McNeal, who gave me the precious opportunity to do research at Stanford University in 1990 and 1991.

I owe great thanks to Prof. Michael Mihatsch, Dr. Holger Moch, Mrs. Rita Epper, and Mrs. Hedwig Weisskopf for careful processing of the radical prostatectomy specimens. Prof. Jakob Roth from the Department of Radiological Physics performed statistical analysis. PD Dr. Franz Hering, Dr. Stephane Rohner, and Mrs. Sandra Kohler helped significantly with follow-up of patients.

Part of this work was supported by the Swiss Urological Association, the Swiss National Science Foundation, and the Richard M. Lucas Foundation (Stanford). Funding for this publication was mainly provided by Hoffmann La Roche Inc., Basel, Switzerland, Ferring AG, Duebendorf and Pharmacia, Duebendorf, Switzerland.

Last, but not least, I would like to thank my parents Emil and Margrit Schmid for their continuous support, and Gaby Zwetsch for our fabulous friendship.

GPSR Compliance

The European Union's (EU) General Product Safety Regulation (GPSR) is a set of rules that requires consumer products to be safe and our obligations to ensure this.

If you have any concerns about our products, you can contact us on ProductSafety@springernature.com

In case Publisher is established outside the EU, the EU authorized representative is:

Springer Nature Customer Service Center GmbH
Europaplatz 3
69115 Heidelberg, Germany

Batch number: 10577969

Printed by Printforce, the Netherlands